RADIOLOGY

Inside Out

DR. VIJAYASHREE GADVE

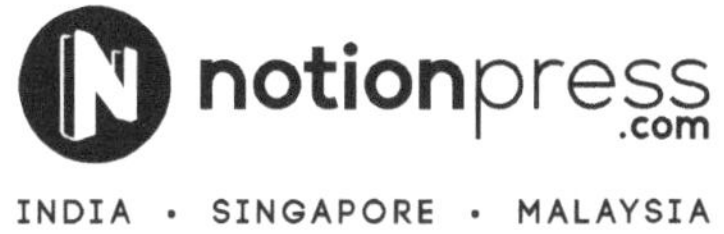

INDIA • SINGAPORE • MALAYSIA

ISBN

Paperback 979-8-89632-969-5
Hardcase 979-8-89724-596-3

CONTENTS

ABOUT THE AUTHOR

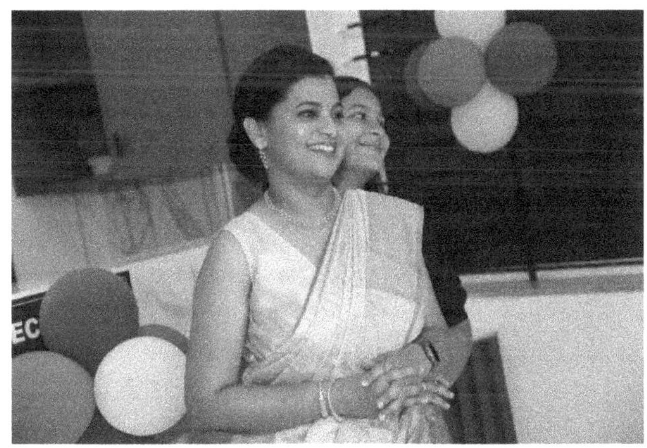

DR. VIJAYASHREE A.GADVE.

MBBS – BLDEA MEDICAL COLLEGE, VIJAYPUR, KARNATAK.

DMRD – KLE'S JN MEDICAL COLLEGE, BELGAUM, KARNATAK.

FELLOW IN USG & COLOUR DOPPLER - SETH G S MEDICAL COLLEGE & KEM HOSPITAL, MUMBAI.

A passionate Radiologist, born and raised in Karnataka, now practicing in Maharashtra while managing another center in Karnataka.

Professionally focused on Fetal medicine, Pediatric & Female Imaging, Sono-Mammography and Color Doppler studies, the author is also deeply committed to community health.

They actively pursue opportunities to conduct programs on breast cancer and Mother-and-Child care.

Beyond their professional endeavors, they enjoy reading, traveling, drawing, occasional cooking, trekking, making new friends, watching movies, and living life to the fullest.

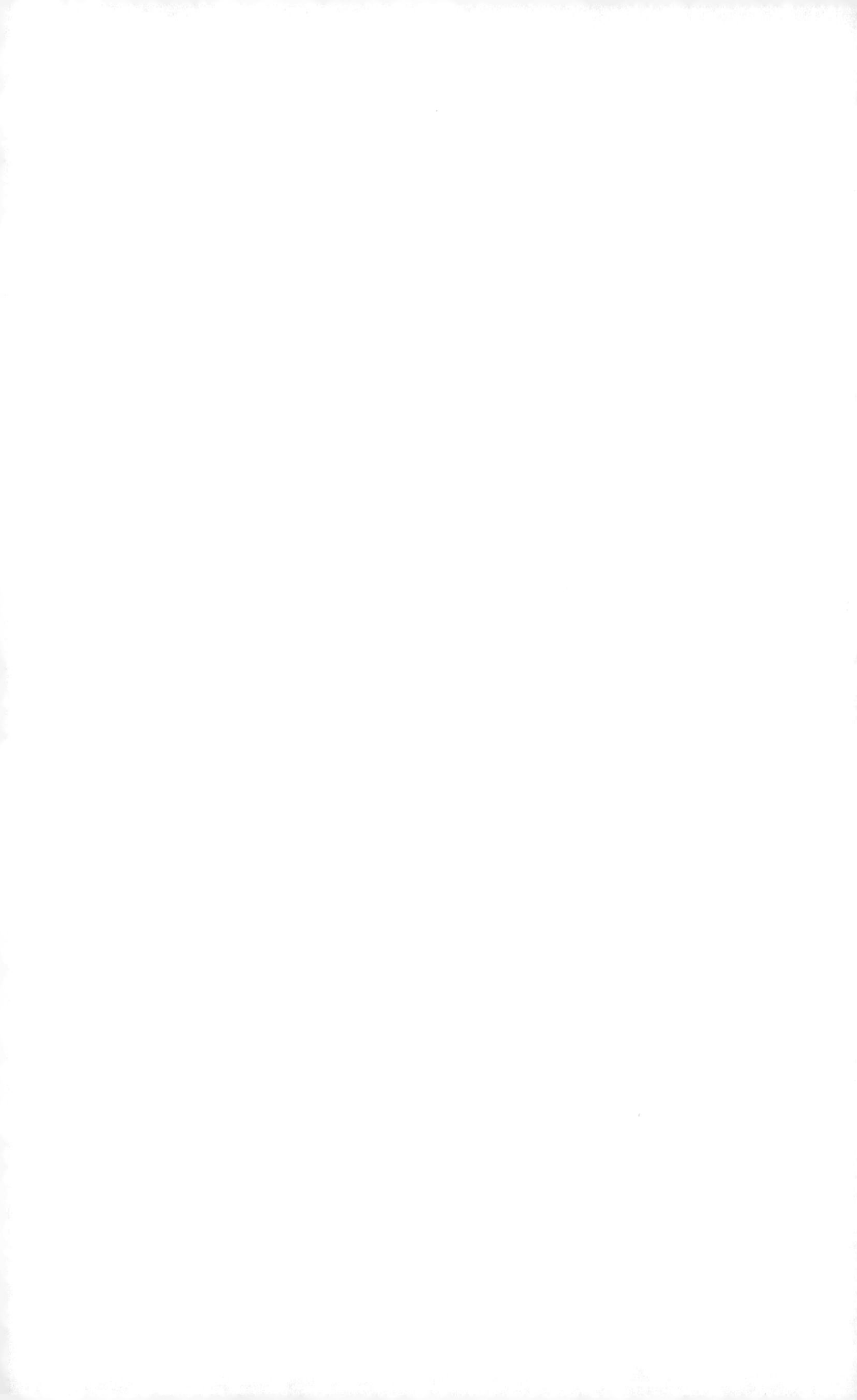

FOREWORDS

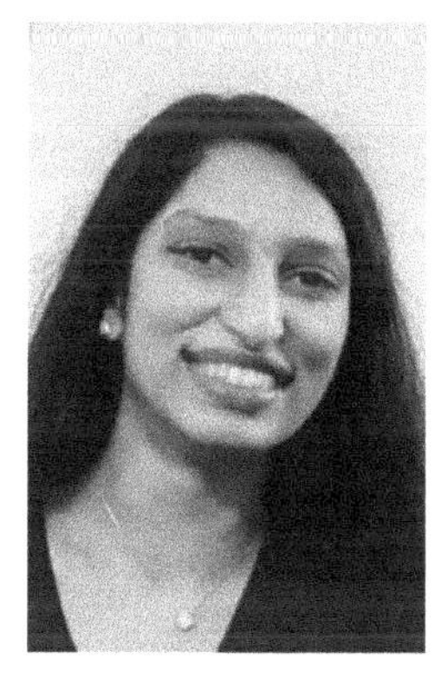

'Inside Out' by the dynamic Dr. Vijayashree Gadve is an absolutely fantastic handbook about the world of radiology! This wonderfully written book introduces the reader to the basics of radiology, an integral field of medicine, that all of us encounter in our lives at some time or the other.

Individual chapters enlighten us about the different modalities of imaging used in radiology. Basic physics of each modality, applications (where the particular modality is most useful), patient preparation and technique are beautifully described in a Q & A format.

Simple language, easy-to-understand line diagrams, fun flowcharts, summaries, and lists of Dos & Don'ts make this book perfect for non-doctors and doctors alike!

I thoroughly enjoyed reading this book and re-living the amazing wonder of discovering radiology's marvels! I'm sure you will love reading the book as well and find it immensely useful! Happy reading!

Dr. Rachita Rama Murthy
Consultant Radiologist
Srinivasa Ultrasound Scanning Centre
Bangalore, India

In an age where medical advancements continue to leap forward, it is crucial for the general public to have a clear, accessible understanding of the technologies that impact their healthcare. "Radiology Inside Out" by Dr. Vijayashree A. Gadve aims to do just that. This book opens a window into the fascinating world of radiology, demystifying the complex processes and innovative techniques that underpin modern medical imaging.

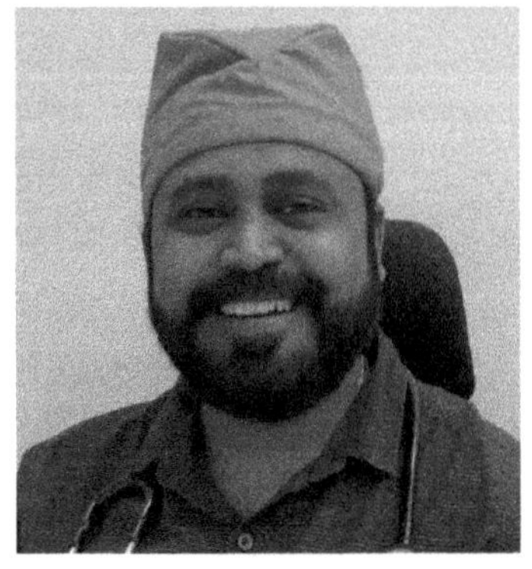

It is with great pleasure that I introduce this remarkable book, "Radiology Inside Out."

As I sit down to pen this foreword, memories of countless X-rays, Echocardiography, MRI scans, and ultrasound images flood my mind. But more importantly, I am reminded of the brilliant radiologist who has authored this invaluable guide: Dr. Vijayashree Gadve.

Radiology plays a pivotal role in diagnosing and managing countless health conditions, yet its workings often remain obscure to those outside the field. Dr. Gadve's work not only clarifies these intricacies but also highlights the profound impact that radiology has on patient care. Her insights will undoubtedly help readers appreciate the critical importance of this speciality in the medical landscape.

It is an honor to write the foreword for this publication. With over 14 years of experience in the field of medicine, I have witnessed firsthand the transformative power of radiological advancements.

Dr. Gadve's dedication to bridging the gap between medical professionals and the public is both commendable and necessary. Her ability to present complex information in an engaging and understandable manner makes this book a valuable resource for anyone seeking to understand the inner workings of medical imaging.

Together, we celebrated victories—the early detection of a malignancy,Heart diseases, the timely diagnosis of a rare congenital anomaly. But we also faced defeats—the moments when shadows eluded us, slipping through our fingers like smoke. Yet even in those moments, Vijayashree's determination never wavered. She would return the next day, eyes bright with resolve, ready to tackle the enigma anew.

I invite you to delve into this enlightening read and discover the extraordinary world of radiology through the expert lens of Dr. Vijayashree A. Gadve. This book is not just an educational journey; it is a testament to the relentless pursuit of knowledge and the unwavering commitment to improving patient care.

So, as you turn these pages, remember that you hold more than a guidebook. You hold a torch—one that illuminates the path toward health, knowledge, and compassion. Whether you're a patient awaiting results or a curious soul seeking insight, "Radiology Inside Out" invites you to peer beyond the surface, to see the world through the eyes of a radiologist.

Thank you, Dr. Vijayashree, for your unwavering commitment. Your hard work, keen eye, and compassionate heart have left an indelible mark on our profession. And to our readers, may this book empower you to decode the shadows—to find not just diagnoses, but also hope.

Warm regards,

DR. RAHUL WARE,
CONSULTING PHYSICIAN. M.D (MEDICINE)
SHREE HOSPITAL , VITA , MAHARASHTRA

This the world behind curtains. Yes, Radiology, as the author calls it 'detective' is an interesting science. As a lay person you must have always wondered, what happens behind the scans? How does all doctors send patients to Radiologists and then get correct diagnosis. Radiology is the guide light for a clinician. This book is designed to empower the common man with the knowledge of how modalities work.

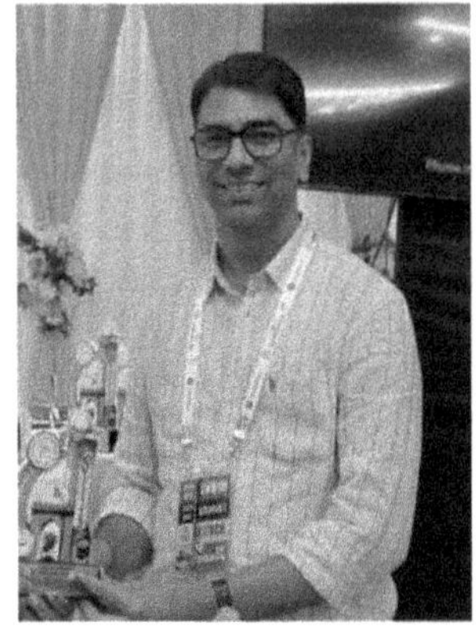

As the reader progress through the chapters, you will realise that author has made it simple to understand most of the aspects. The book explains principles, procedures and applications of each modality. The book explains how the tests are used and are complimentary for diagnosing disease. The book will help reader to reduce the anxiety about these tests, have a better underunderstanding about the same when a doctor prescribes it, ask relevant doubts to the clinician and take conscious decisions considering pros and cons of a modality.

Authors dedication to radiology, sense of social responsibility and passion towards educating everyone, makes this book essential for everyone.

This book is a valuable resource for acting as a guide light in the sea of healthcare system and guide you with clarity and confidence.

Unwavering efforts of Dr. Vijayshree towards Radiology education has made us get connected.

DR DHANANJAY GHONGADE
DNB RADIOLOGY
SAI SCANS, KOLHAPUR
MAHARASHTRA

It is with great pleasure that I hold in my hands this impressive manuscript of Radiology : Inside out.

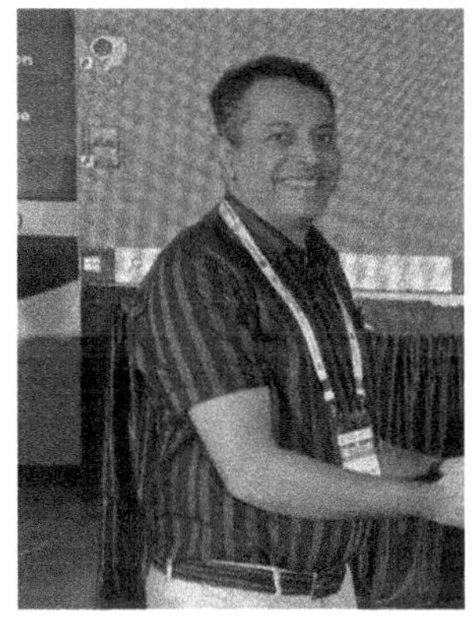

Radiology department is one of the commonest department visited by every patient after general physician and surgeons office. Lot of different machines with wide spectrum of investigations on each can be scary for the patients and their close relatives.

This book will surely provide a primer of Radiology Doctors, Paramedics, various radiological investigations as well as the machines used in this department, knowing which will significantly decrease the pre-checkup anxiety of each one. This book is well structured and is presented in easy to understand chapters with the most up to date knowledge in this complicated radiology field.

Simple language, indicative diagrams, neat layouts and eye-catching animations further facilitate to the understanding of the content of the book.

Short but complete information will surely be helpful to the departmental beneficiaries and will further help the treating doctors' team to convince the WHY, HOW, WHERE, and WHEN of each required investigation for the particular disease of that patient.

I congratulate the author of this book for such an incredible product.

I cannot wait to get my inscribed copy soon.

Dr. Bharat Mudalgi
M.B.B.S, M.D
Consultant Radiologist.
Akshay Diagnostic Center and Sai Scans, Sangli.

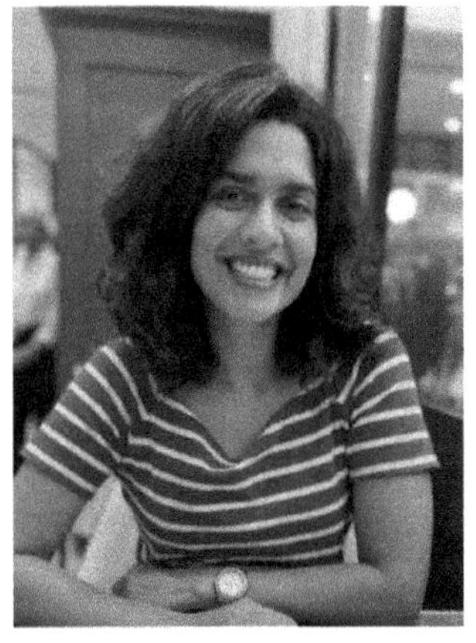

"Radiology Inside Out" is a breath of fresh air. It simplifies complex concepts, making them accessible to readers from all backgrounds and non-medicos such as myself. The book offers a comprehensive overview of radiology, from its historical roots to the latest advancements in imaging technology.

One of the most impressive aspects of this book is its ability to demystify the various imaging modalities. Whether it's X-rays, MRIs, ultrasounds or CT scans, the author explains how these technologies work and what kind of information they provide. The lucid explanations and clear illustrations make it easy to understand even the most intricate details.

Interventional radiology, a field that often remains shrouded in mystery, is also explored in depth. Dr. Vijayshree provides a fascinating glimpse into the world of minimally invasive procedures, highlighting the significant impact of this specialty on modern medicine.

In conclusion, "Radiology Inside Out" is a valuable resource for anyone seeking to understand the intricacies of medical imaging. It's a testament to the author's ability to communicate complex scientific concepts in a clear and engaging manner. Whether you're a curious layperson or a healthcare professional, this book offers a wealth of knowledge and insights.

ESHA SHAH, BE IN ARCHITECT

CHAPTER 1

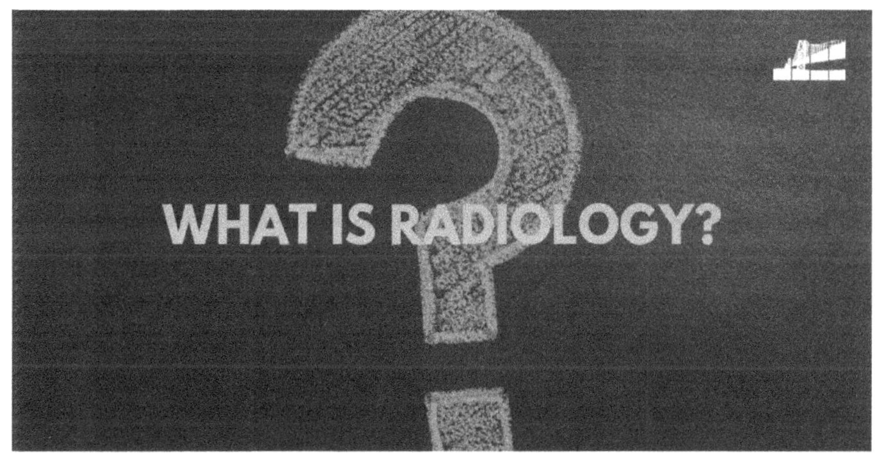

Imagine walking into a room where you can see what's happening inside without opening it up. This is the magic of radiology , a field of medicine that allows us to peer inside the human body without a single cut.

It's the silent hero that helps doctors visualize the unseen and make informed decisions about treatment.

In this book, we'll embark on a journey through the fascinating world of Radiology.

We'll explore how different imaging technologies work, discover how they're used to diagnose a wide range of conditions, and understand the impact they have on patient care.

Whether you're a curious reader, a patient preparing for an imaging procedure, or someone interested in the marvels of medical technology, this book will open your eyes to the incredible power of Radiology.

Think of radiology as a detective in the world of Medicine. Just as a detective uses clues to solve mysteries, Radiologists use images to uncover hidden problems within the body.

FEW COMMON REAL LIFE STORIES WHICH YOU COME ACROSS ON DAILY BASIS

SCENARIO 1

Malati , a 45-year-old school teacher, began experiencing persistent headaches. After a detailed assessment, her doctor recommended an MRI to check for any abnormalities in her Brain. Malati was nervous but found that the process was less complicated than she had expected. The MRI revealed a benign tumour, which was successfully treated.

SCENARIO 2

A 62-year-old man with continuous cough, loss of weight, appetite and feeling short of breath. After preliminary X ray CT scan of chest was used to identify the tumor's size and location, leading to a successful surgical intervention.

SCENARIO 3

Now story of a young cricketer who sustained a knee injury. Initial X-rays showed no fractures, but an MRI revealed a torn ligament. The detailed images guided the treatment plan, which included surgery and physical therapy.

"WALKTHROUGH OF A RADIOLOGY DEPARTMENT"

Here is the gross overview , how a diagnostic centre looks like !

Bird's eye view of my own diagnostic centre...,

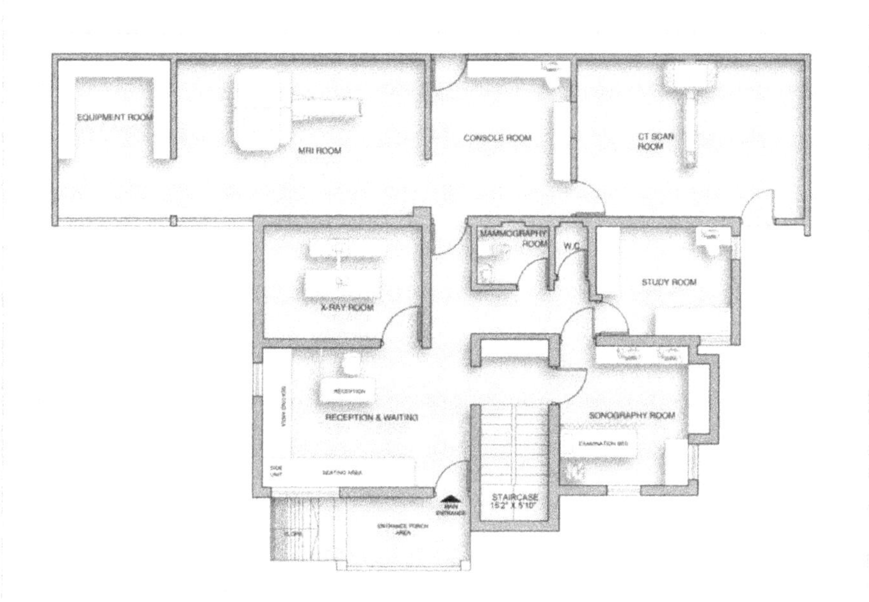

ANVI DIAGNOSTIC IMAGING , SANGLI
PC : ARCHITECT AJINKYA MAHABAL

Now let's Meet the Radiology Team

Roles Explained:

Radiologist

The doctor who looks at the pictures and figures out what's going on inside your body!

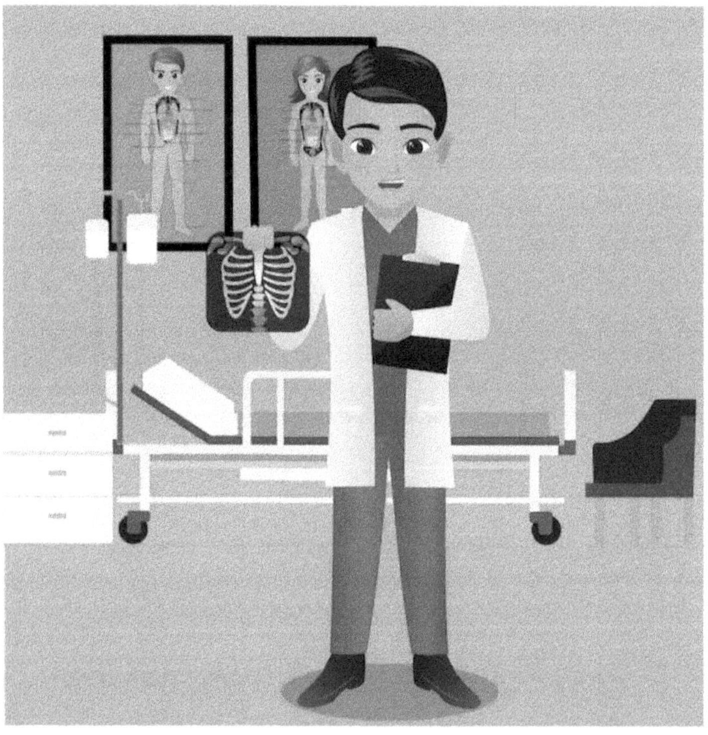

Radiology Technician:

This person helps take the pictures.

They help you lie down, stay still and feel comfortable.

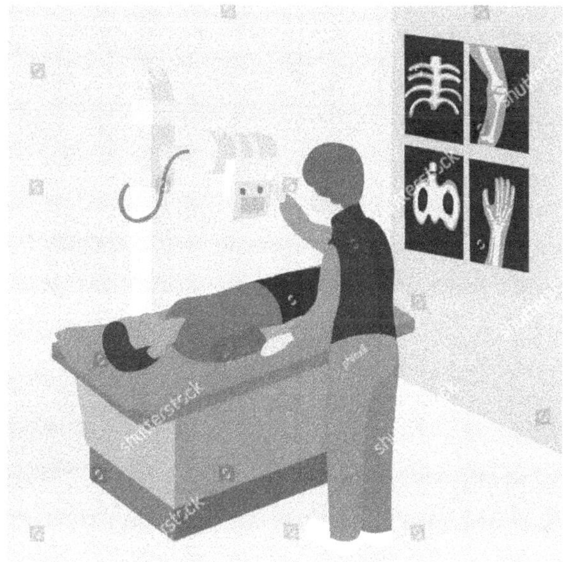

Nurse:

The nurse is there to make sure you're feeling okay and to explain everything that's going to happen.

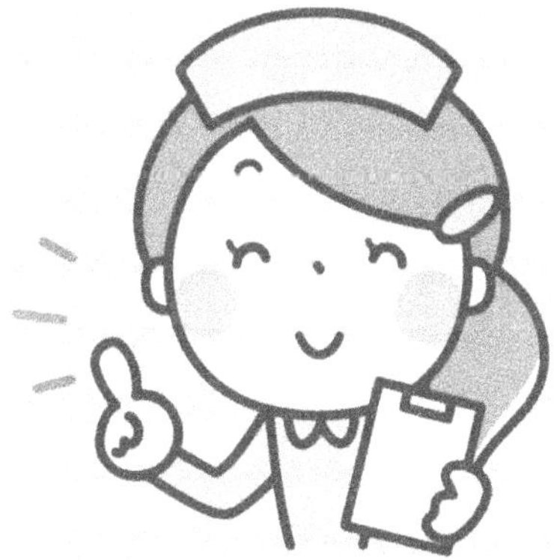

Exploring the Imaging Machines

X-Ray Machine

An X-ray machine is a device that uses invisible rays of high-energy light to create images of the inside of the body, helping doctors see bones, organs, and tissues.

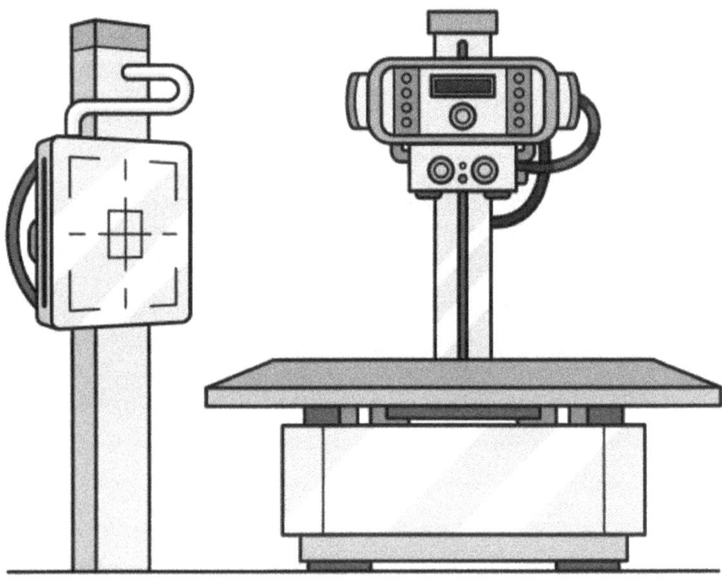

CT Scanner

The CT machine is like a giant doughnut you lie down inside!

It takes lots of pictures of your body from different angles and makes a 3D image.

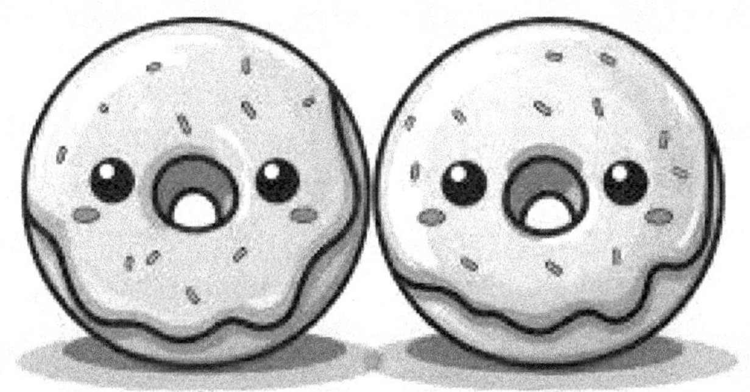

MRI Machine

An MRI machine looks like a big tunnel. You lie down and stay still, and it uses magnets to take super-detailed pictures of your insides. It's great for looking at muscles and the brain.

- **Important Fact: MRIs don't use radiation, just magnets, and sound waves !**

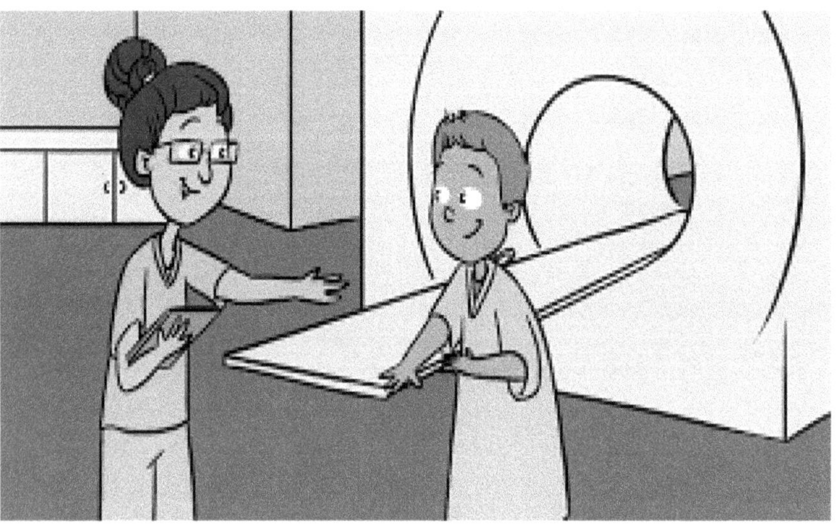

Ultrasound Machine:

This machine uses sound waves to look inside your body. The Sonologist puts some cool gel on your skin and then moves a little camera over it. You can even see the picture on the screen!

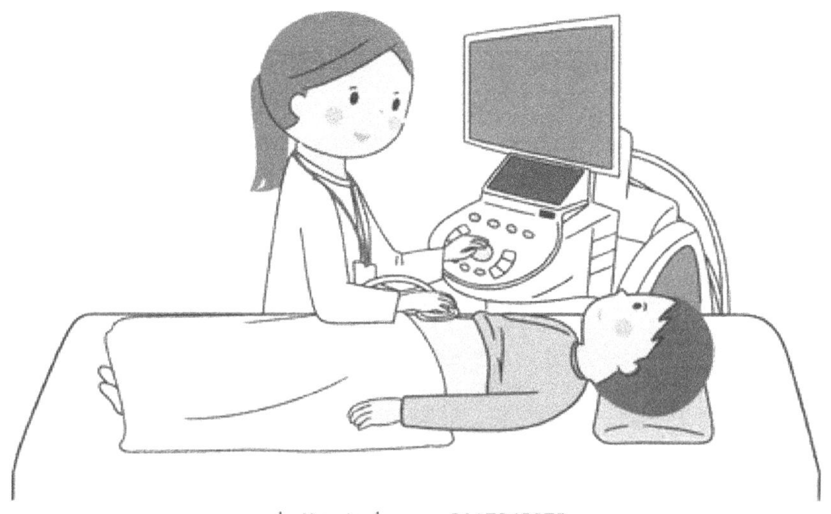

Safety First!

In the radiology department, we make sure you're super safe! Sometimes you might wear a heavy apron made of lead. It helps protect parts of your body that aren't getting a picture.

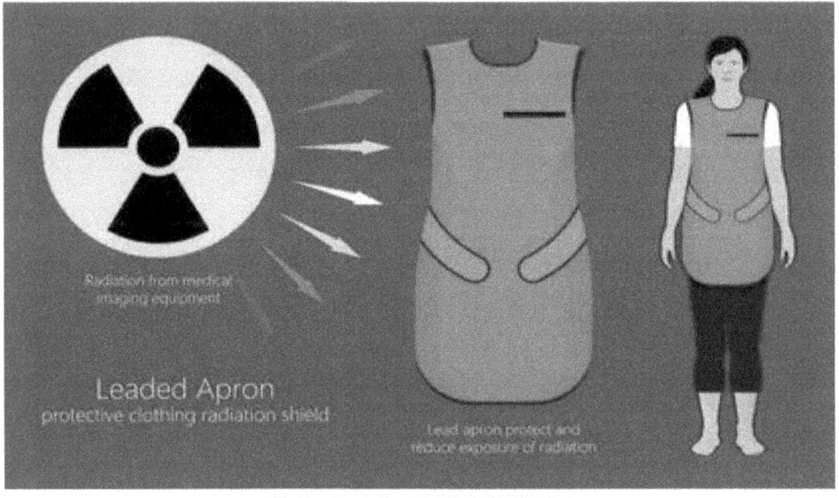

What Happens During the Imaging Test ?

Step-by-Step:

1. **Getting Ready**
2. **Taking the Picture**
3. **Finished!: After the picture is taken, you get to leave, and the Radiologist will look at the images to figure out what's happening inside your body.**

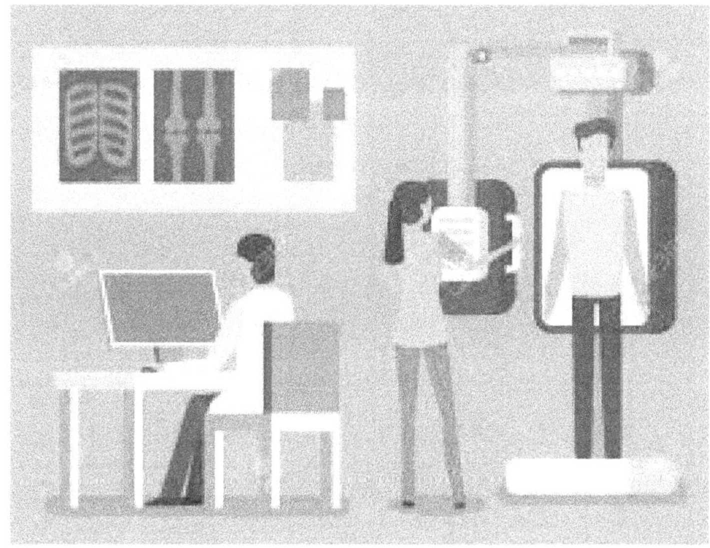

Cool Pictures from the Inside

After the pictures are taken, the radiologist looks at them on a computer. These pictures show what's going on inside your body.

Sometimes radiologists can see things that are super tiny, even smaller than a grain of rice !

They will prepare report out of that and will be given to you after certain time with full verification.

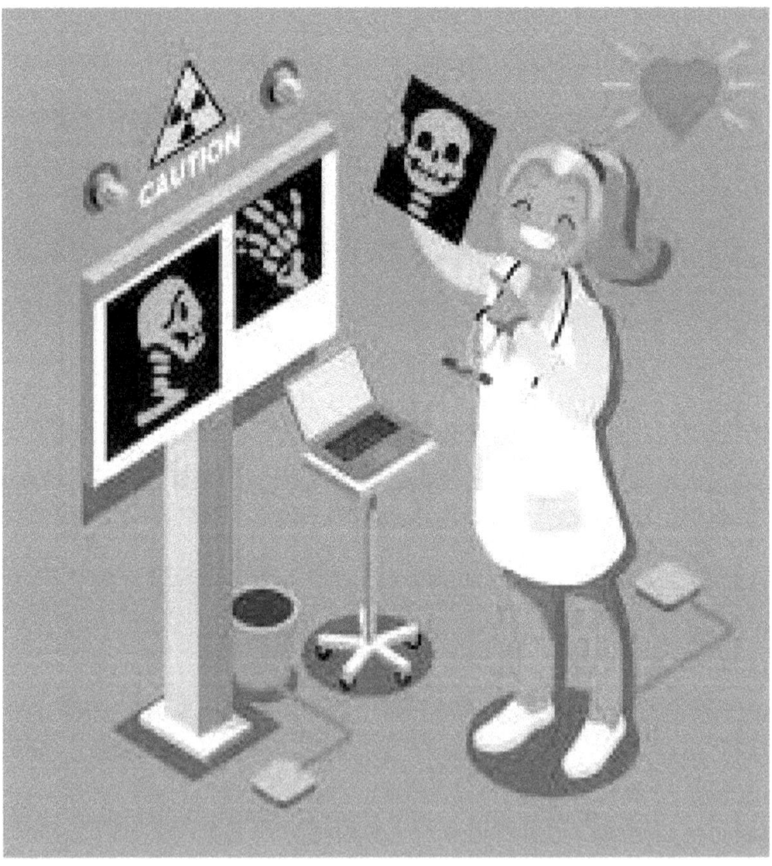

CHAPTER 2

GLOSSARY OF RADIOLOGY TERMS

1. **X-ray:** A type of radiation used to create images of inside of the body. X-rays can help diagnose fractures, infections, and other conditions.
2. **CT Scan** (Computed Tomography Scan): A medical imaging technique that uses a series of X-ray images taken from different angles and combines them to create cross-sectional images of the body.
3. **MRI** (Magnetic Resonance Imaging): A technique that uses strong magnets and radio waves to create detailed images of organs and tissues inside the body, particularly useful for soft tissues.
4. **Ultrasound:** An imaging method that uses high-frequency sound waves to create images of organs and structures inside the body. It is often used for monitoring pregnancies and examining soft tissues.
5. **Radiologist:** A medical doctor who specializes in interpreting medical images, such as X-rays, CT scans, MRIs, and ultrasounds.
6. **Contrast Agent:** A substance used to improve the visibility of internal structures in imaging tests. It can be swallowed, injected, or inserted into the body depending on the type of scan.

7. **Fluoroscopy:** An imaging technique that uses X-rays to obtain real-time moving images of the inside of the body, often used to guide procedures like catheter insertions.
8. **PET Scan** (Positron Emission Tomography): A type of imaging test that uses a small amount of radioactive material to show how organs and tissues are functioning. It is often used in cancer diagnosis and treatment.
9. **Biopsy:** A procedure to remove a small sample of tissue for examination under a microscope. Imaging techniques like ultrasound or CT can guide the biopsy.
10. **Mammogram:** An X-ray image of the breast used to screen for breast cancer and other abnormalities.
11. **Radiopaque:** Refers to materials that block X-rays and appear white on X-ray images, such as bones or certain contrast agents.
12. **Radiolucent:** Refers to materials that allow X-rays to pass through and appear dark on X-ray images, such as air or fluids.
13. **Echo**: Short for echocardiogram, this is an ultrasound test specifically for viewing the heart and its function.
14. **Tomography:** An imaging technique that creates detailed cross-sectional images of the body, such as those from CT or PET scans.
15. **Imaging:** The process of creating visual representations of the interior of a body for clinical analysis and medical intervention.

16. **Angiogram:** An imaging test that uses X-rays and contrast dye to visualize blood vessels and check for blockages or abnormalities.

17. **Radiation:** Energy emitted in the form of waves or particles, used in X-rays and other imaging techniques to create images of the body.

18. **Dose:** The amount of radiation exposure a person receives during an imaging procedure.

19. **Artifact:** An error or distortion in an image that does not represent the actual anatomy or pathology, often caused by movement or technical factors.

20. **Scan:** A general term for a medical imaging procedure, such as X-ray, CT scan, or MRI.

This glossary can help demystify the terminology and make Radiology more accessible to readers.

CHAPTER 3

DO IT YOURSELF TO UNDERSTAND RADIOLOGY

"Do It Yourself (DIY) to Understand Radiology" section will provide fun, easy experiments or activities that readers can do at home to help them grasp key radiology concepts.

Here are some DIY ideas:

1. **X-ray Simulation with Flashlight and Objects**
   - **Objective**: Show how X-rays pass through certain materials but not others, simulating how Radiologists see bones and dense tissues.
   - **Materials**:
     - Flashlight (X-ray beam)
     - Various objects (paper, plastic, metal, cardboard)
     - White sheet or thin fabric (to act as a "screen")
   - **Instructions**:
     1. Shine the flashlight through different objects onto the sheet.
     2. Observe how dense objects (like metal) block more light, just as bones block X-rays.
     3. Explain that softer tissues, like skin and muscles, appear lighter on X-rays, just like the paper or fabric lets more light through.

- **Concept**: This activity helps visualize how different densities in the body create X-ray images.

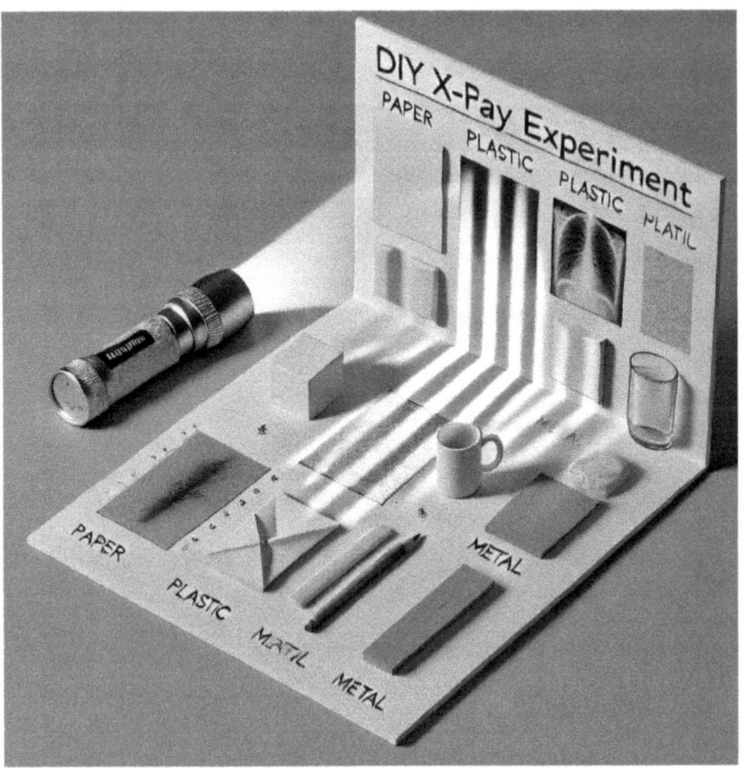

2. **Create Your Own "Ultrasound"**

- **Objective**: Demonstrate how sound waves can be used to create images, similar to how ultrasound uses sound to visualize inside the body.
- **Materials**:
    - Small speaker or buzzer
    - Water
    - Plastic wrap or a balloon filled with water
    - A small object (like a toy or coin) placed inside the water-filled balloon

- **Instructions**:
    1. Place the object inside the water balloon and cover it tightly with plastic wrap.
    2. Put the small speaker next to the balloon, sending vibrations into the water.
    3. Watch the ripples and think of them as sound waves bouncing off the object inside, showing where it is.
- **Concept**: Ultrasound waves bounce off structures inside the body (like the object in the balloon) and the machine translates these echoes into an image.

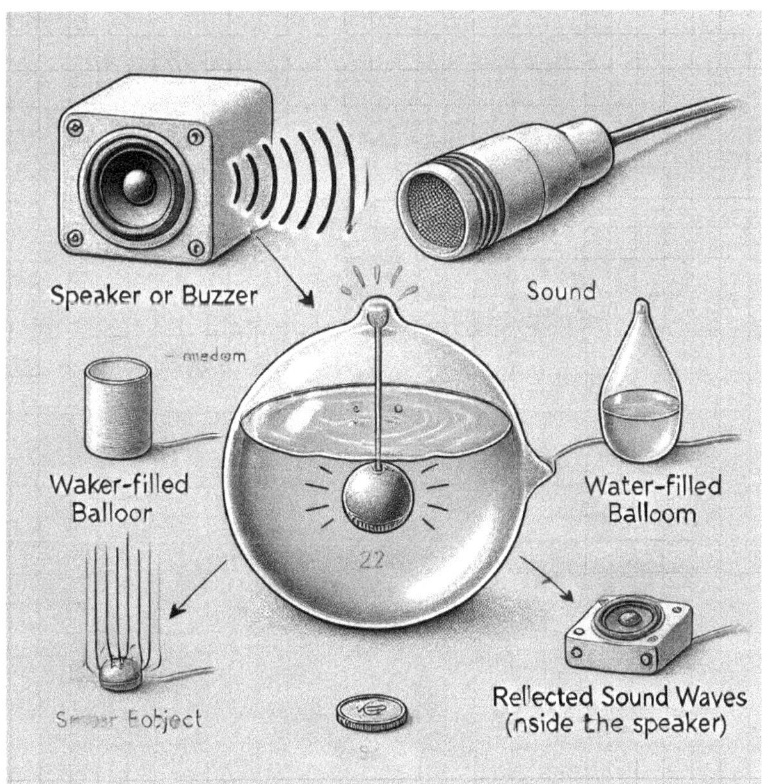

3. **MRI with a Magnet and Iron Filings**

- **Objective**: Understand the concept of magnetic resonance and how MRI uses strong magnets to produce images.
- **Materials**:
  - Magnet
  - Iron filings (or small metal objects like paper clips)
  - Clear plastic sheet or paper
- **Instructions**:
  1. Place the clear sheet over the magnet and sprinkle iron filings or small metal objects on top.
  2. Watch how the filings align with the magnetic field.
  3. Explain that MRI uses strong magnetic fields to align water molecules in the body, and when the magnetic field is turned off, the molecules release energy that the MRI scanner detects and converts into images.
- **Concept**: This demonstrates how magnetic fields can be used to "see" patterns, similar to how MRI scans create images of tissues.

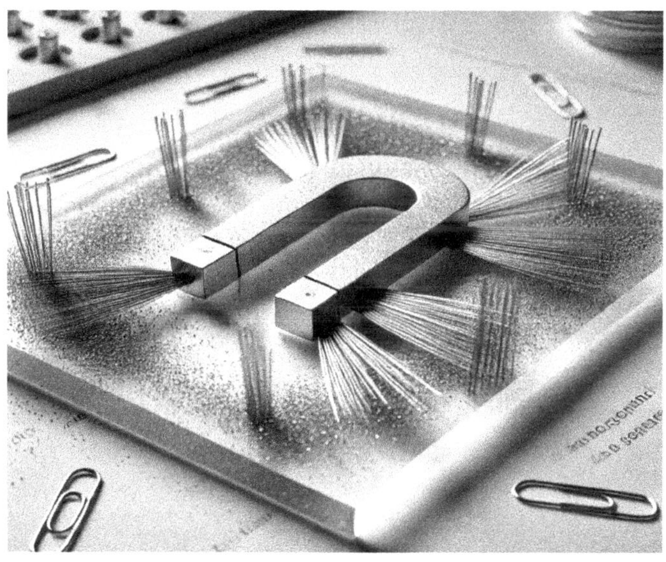

4. **Radiation Comparison Chart Using Everyday Items**
    - **Objective**: Help readers understand different levels of radiation exposure using relatable items.
    - **Materials**:
        - Common household items like a banana, smoke detector, granite countertop (each emits small amounts of radiation).
        - Chart paper and stickers.
    - **Instructions**:
        1. Research and create a chart showing how much radiation each item emits, comparing it to medical imaging (e.g., a banana emits about 0.1 microsieverts, while a chest X-ray is about 100 microsieverts).

2. Use stickers or draw bars to compare the radiation levels of common objects to that of X-rays, CT scans and MRIs.

- **Concept**: Readers learn that many everyday items emit small amounts of radiation, helping them understand that medical imaging is often within safe levels.

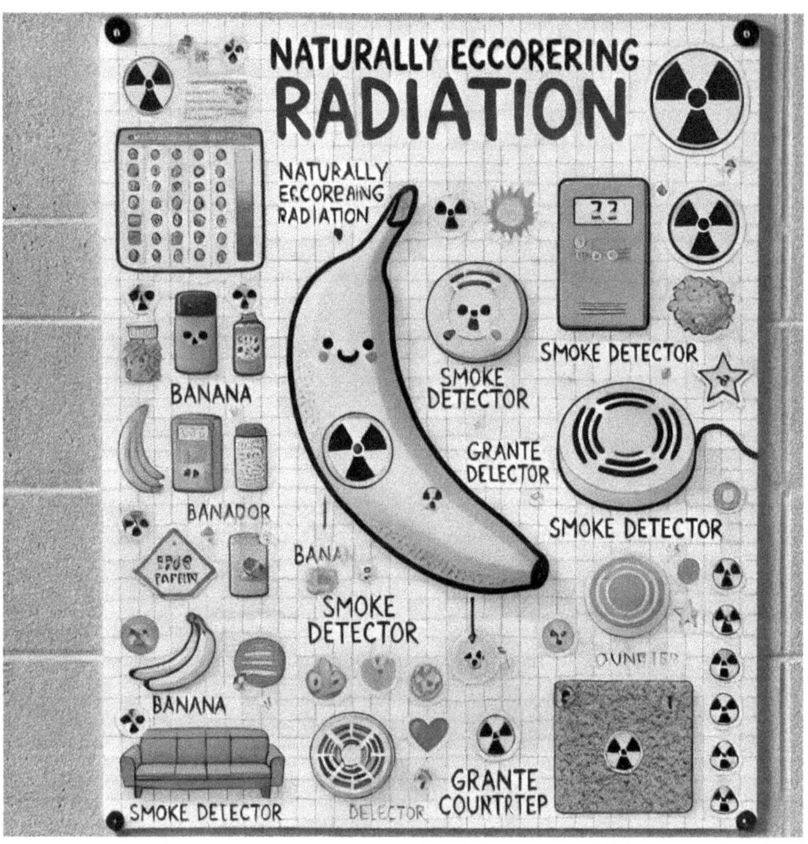

5. **Build a Simple "Radiology Department" at Home**

- **Objective**: Teach the steps of radiology processes and roles in a fun, play-acting way.

- **Materials**:
    - Printouts or drawings of medical imaging machines (X-ray, CT scanner, ultrasound).
    - Cardboard boxes to build mock machines.
    - Role-playing cards for radiologists, technicians, and patients.

- **Instructions**:
    - Set up a mini "Radiology department" at home with homemade imaging machines.
    - Have family members or friends take turns being the Radiologist, Technician, or Patient.
    - Walk through a simple scenario (e.g., Diagnosing a broken arm using a pretend X-ray).

- **Concept**: Helps kids and adults understand the workflow of a Radiology department, demystifying what happens behind the scenes.

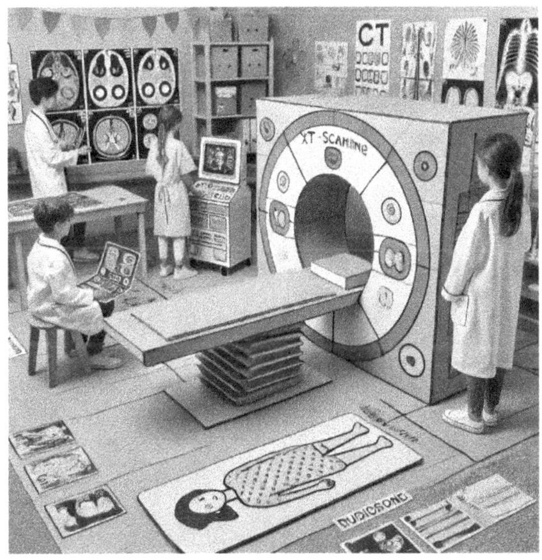

6. **Radiation Shielding Experiment**

   - **Objective**: Show how different materials can block radiation, similar to how lead aprons protect patients during X-rays.
   - **Materials**:
     - Flashlight (as a "radiation source").
     - Different materials (foil, plastic, cloth, paper).
   - **Instructions**:
     1. Shine the flashlight through each material and observe how much light passes through.
     2. Compare this to how radiation penetrates the body, with denser materials like lead blocking more radiation (just like foil blocks more light).

- **Concept**: Teaches the concept of radiation protection and the importance of shielding during imaging.

These hands-on activities can make radiology concepts easier to understand while making the learning process fun

CHAPTER 4

The Fascinating History of Radiology: From X-rays to AI

Radiology, a field often associated with high-tech images and life-saving diagnoses, has a history filled with fascinating milestones, remarkable discoveries, and surprising stories.

Here are some key points and fun facts to include in a chapter dedicated to the history of radiology:

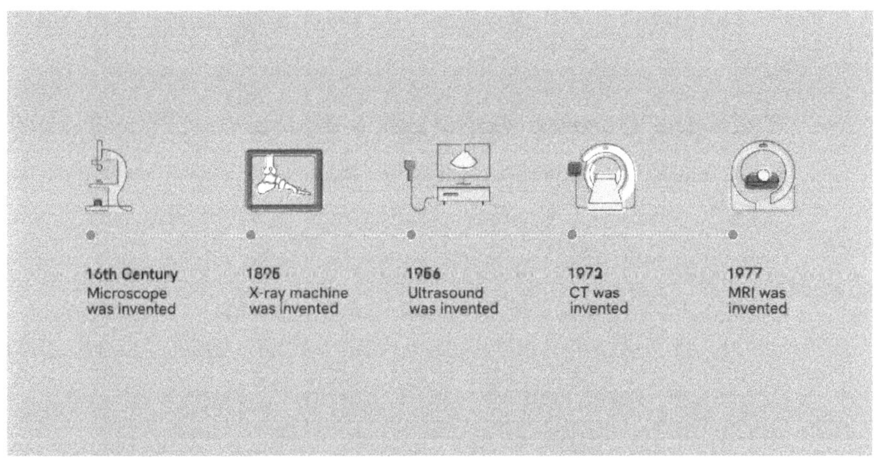

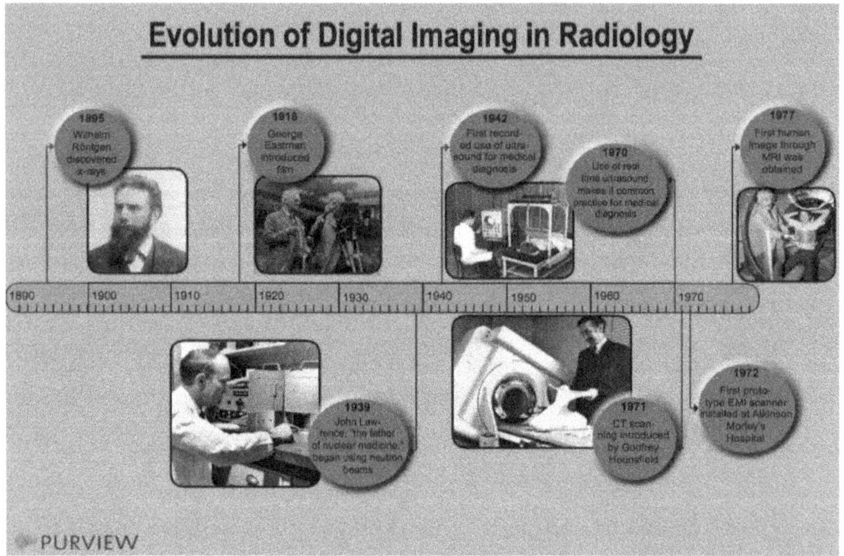

1. **The Discovery of X-rays: A Serendipitous Accident (1895)**

   - **Wilhelm Conrad Roentgen's Discovery**: The history of radiology begins with a monumental accident in 1895. Wilhelm Conrad Roentgen, a German physicist, was experimenting with cathode rays when he noticed a mysterious glow on a nearby screen. It turned out he had discovered a new type of ray that could pass through solid objects and create shadowy images of bones – he called these "X-rays," where "X" represented the unknown.

   - **First X-ray Image**: Roentgen's first X-ray image was of his wife's hand, revealing her bones and wedding ring. When she saw it, she reportedly exclaimed, "I have seen my death!" The image became iconic, and Roentgen's discovery changed medicine forever.

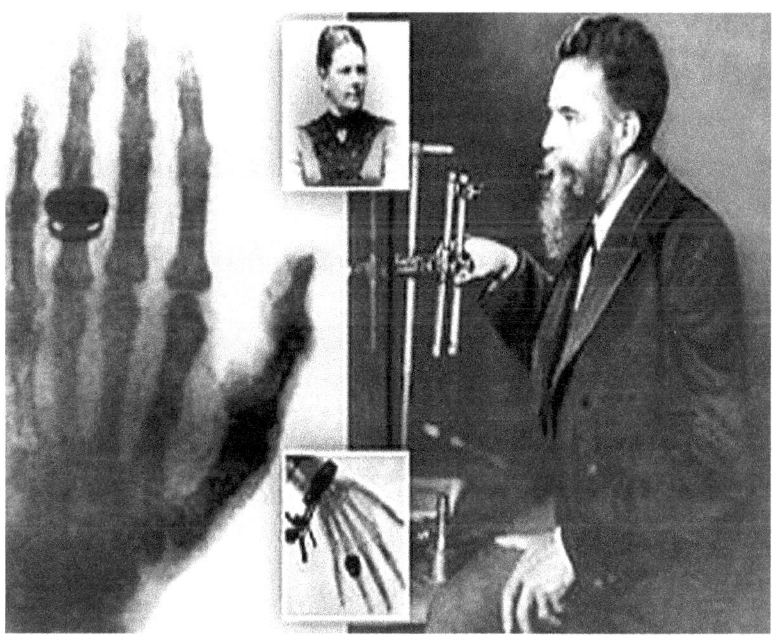

2. **The Rise of Medical Imaging (Early 1900s)**

   - **X-rays in Medicine**: Soon after Roentgen's discovery, X-rays were quickly adopted for medical use. Physicians could now look inside the human body without making a single incision! This led to significant improvements in diagnosing fractures, foreign objects, and diseases like tuberculosis.

   - **Marie Curie's Role**: Not only is Marie Curie known for her research on radioactivity, but she also contributed to radiology during World War I. She developed mobile X-ray units (known as "Little Curies") that were used on the battlefield to help doctors treat wounded soldiers.

3. **Fun Fact: Early Radiologists Took Huge Risks**

   - **Dangers of Early X-rays**: In the early days, the harmful effects of X-ray exposure were unknown. Radiologists would often expose themselves to radiation without protection, leading to severe burns, hair loss, and even cancer. Many early pioneers of Radiology, including Thomas Edison's assistant Clarence Dally, suffered from radiation sickness or died from overexposure.

- **Early X-ray Machines in Shoe Stores**: In the 1930s to 1950s, X-ray machines called "fluoroscopes" were used in shoe stores to measure how well shoes fit customers. People would stick their feet into the machines to see the bones of their feet inside the shoes – a practice now known to be dangerous due to excessive radiation exposure!

4. **The Birth of Modern Imaging: Ultrasound, CT, and MRI (1950s-1970s)**

- **Ultrasound**: In the 1950s, ultrasound technology was introduced, using high-frequency sound waves to create images of soft tissues. Initially used for industrial purposes, ultrasound revolutionized prenatal care, allowing doctors to see the developing fetus inside the womb for the first time.

- **CT Scans**: In 1972, Sir Godfrey Hounsfield and Dr. Allan Cormack developed the first Computed Tomography (CT) scanner. CT scans produce detailed, cross-sectional images of the body, combining X-rays and computer technology. Hounsfield's invention earned him a Nobel Prize in Medicine.

- **MRI**: Magnetic Resonance Imaging (MRI) was developed in the 1970s and quickly became one of the most powerful tools in Radiology. Unlike X-rays or CT scans, MRIs use powerful magnets and radio waves to create highly detailed images of organs, tissues, and even the brain. Dr. Raymond Damadian was instrumental in the development of MRI technology.

5. **Fun Fact: MRIs and Nobel Prize Controversy**

   - **Nobel Prize Snub**: Despite Dr. Raymond Damadian's critical role in developing MRI technology, he was controversially excluded when the Nobel Prize in Medicine was awarded in 2003 to Paul Lauterbur and Peter Mansfield, who refined the technology. This sparked outrage in the scientific community, as many believed Damadian's contribution was equally deserving.

6. **Radiology Goes Digital (1980s-Present)**

   - **Digital Imaging**: The 1980s and 1990s saw a shift from traditional film-based radiology to digital imaging, allowing for faster, more accurate, and easily shareable images. PACS (Picture Archiving and Communication Systems) emerged as a tool for storing, retrieving, and viewing medical images digitally.

   - **PET Scans and Nuclear Medicine**: Positron Emission Tomography (PET) scans, introduced in the 1990s, allowed doctors to observe metabolic processes in the body, which is especially useful in cancer diagnosis and neurological conditions.

7. **The Future of Radiology: AI and Beyond**

   - **Artificial Intelligence in Radiology**: Today, artificial intelligence (AI) is revolutionizing radiology by helping radiologists analyze complex scans faster and more accurately. AI algorithms can detect patterns that are invisible to the human eye, assisting in early diagnosis of diseases like cancer and Alzheimer's.

- **3D and Virtual Reality Imaging**: Radiology is also stepping into the world of 3D printing and virtual reality, allowing doctors to print 3D models of organs and tumors or use VR to "walk through" a patient's body before surgery.

8. **Fun Fact: Radiology in Pop Culture**

- **X-rays in Pop Culture**: X-rays have appeared in numerous TV shows and movies. One notable example is the famous X-ray vision of Superman. The concept of seeing through objects, initially a scientific marvel, became a pop culture superpower.
- **Hollywood's Love for MRIs and CTs**: Medical dramas like *House* and *Grey's Anatomy* frequently showcase MRI and CT machines, sometimes dramatically "finding" tumors or other critical issues. These scans have become a storytelling tool for adding tension in medical TV shows.

Conclusion: From Accidents to AI

Radiology has evolved from a fortunate accident in Roentgen's lab to one of the most advanced fields in modern medicine. With innovations like AI, 3D imaging and the continuous refinement of imaging techniques, Radiology remains at the cutting edge of medical science, helping doctors diagnose and treat millions of patients worldwide.

CHAPTER 5

UNDERSTANDING X-RAYS

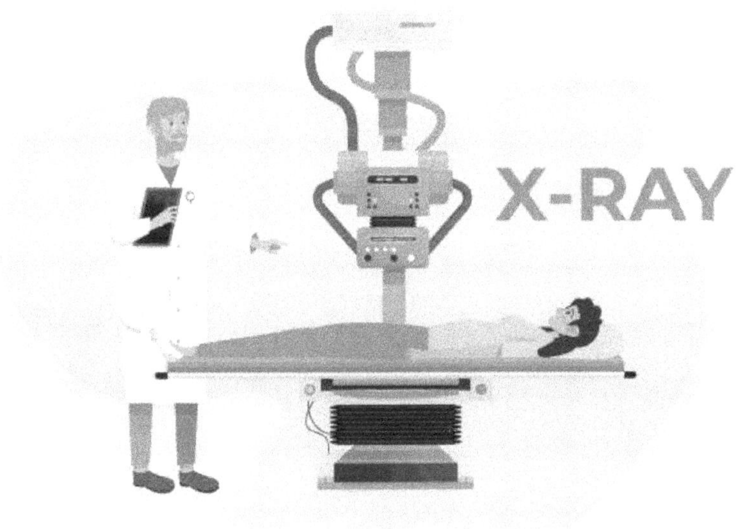

- **How X-rays Work**: A simple explanation of how X-rays use radiation to create images.
- **What Patients Should Expect**: Walk through a typical X-ray procedure.
- **Safety and Risks**: Discuss the minimal risks of X-rays and how medical professionals ensure safety.

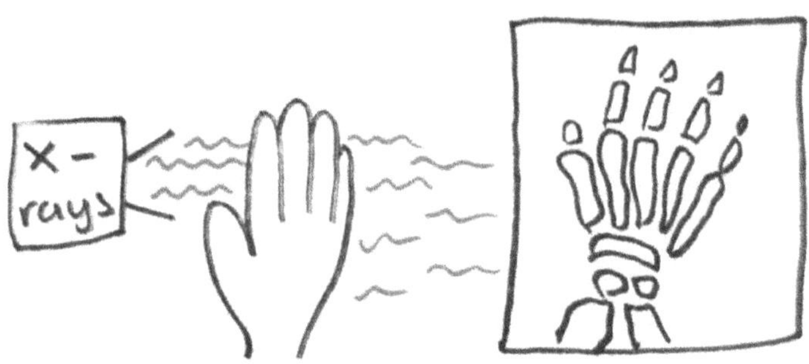

How Do X-rays Work?

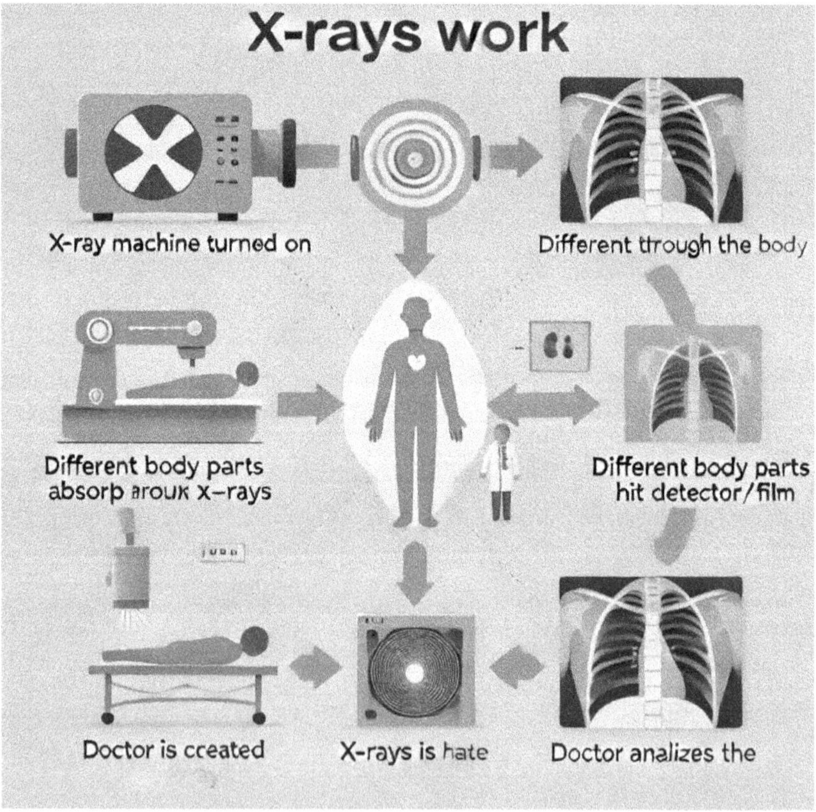

X-rays work

X-ray machine turned on

Different ttrough the body

Different body parts
absorp arouk x–rays

Different body parts
hit detector/film

Doctor is cceated

X-rays is hate

Doctor analizes the

What Happens During an X-ray?

The process of getting an X-ray is quick and painless. Here's what typically happens:

[Check-In] → [Provide Information]

↓

[Change into a Gown]

↓

[Remove Metal Objects]

↓

[Position Yourself]

↓

[Position X-Ray Machine]

↓

[Hold Still]

↓

[Retrieve Personal Items]

↓

[Wait for Results]

↓

[Consult Your Doctor]

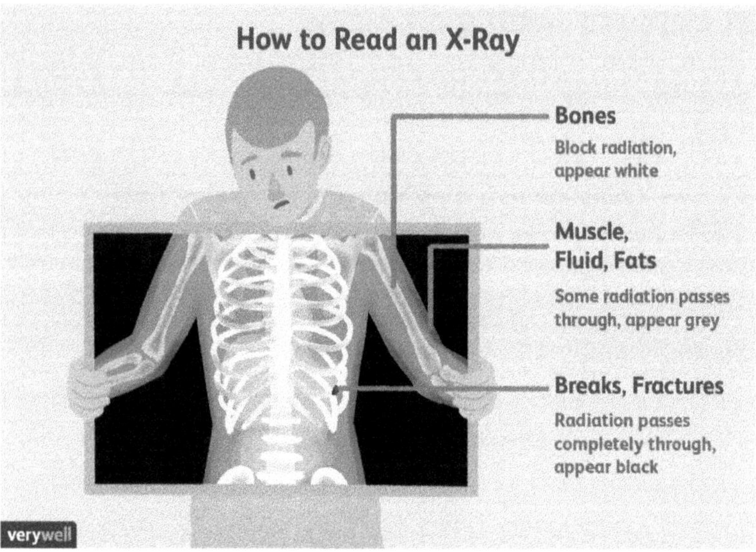

What Are X-rays Used For?

X-rays can help diagnose a variety of conditions and injuries, such as:

- **Bone fractures**: X-rays can quickly show if a bone is broken and how severe the break is.
- **Chest problems**: Doctors use chest X-rays to look at the lungs and heart. They can detect pneumonia, lung tumors, or fluid around the heart.
- **Dental issues**: Dentists often use X-rays to check for cavities or other dental problems.
- **Infections**: Sometimes, X-rays can help detect infections in bones or organs.
- **Joint problems**: X-rays can show arthritis or other issues in the joints.

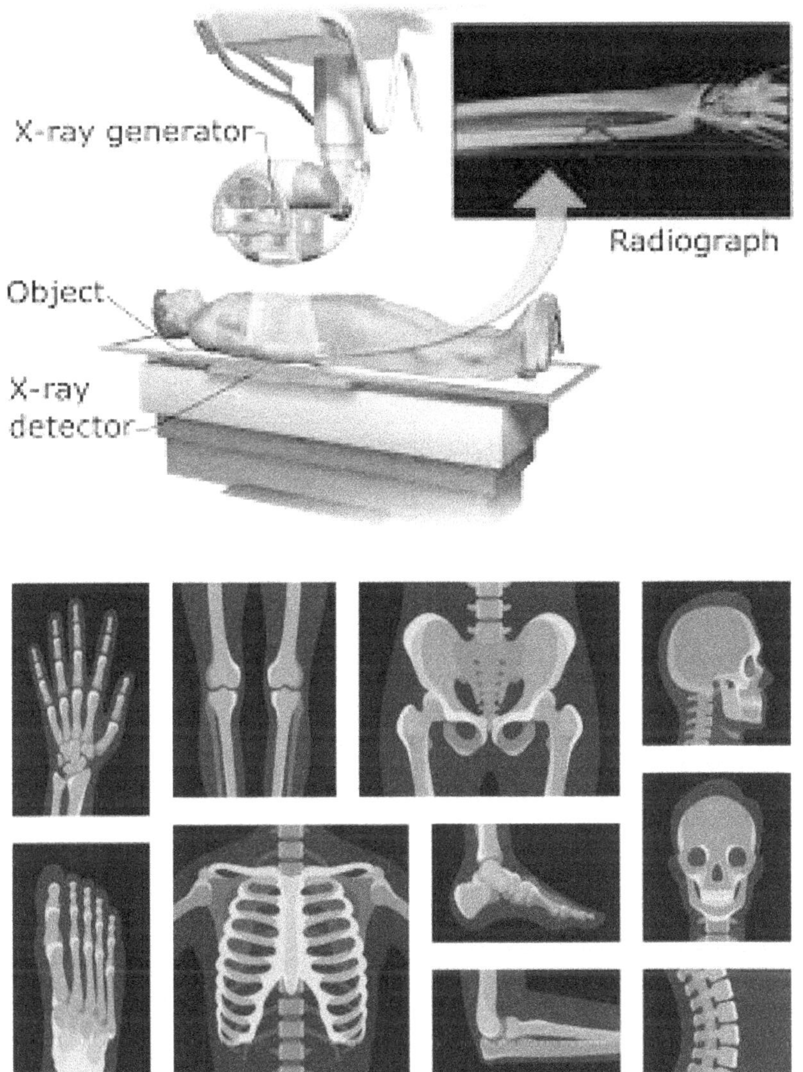

X RAY'S OF VARIOUS PARTS OF BODY

Are X-rays Safe?

For most people, X-rays are safe.

Pregnant women should avoid X-rays unless absolutely necessary, as radiation can pose a risk to the developing baby.

Common Questions About X-rays:

- **Is it dangerous?**
    - X-rays use very small amounts of radiation, and the benefits of diagnosing a medical problem usually far outweigh the risks. For most people, occasional exposure to X-rays is considered safe.
- **Will I feel anything?**
    - No, you won't feel the X-rays themselves. The only discomfort may come from holding a certain position during the imaging.
- **Why do I have to wear a protective shield?**
    - Sometimes, a lead apron is provided to protect certain parts of your body from unnecessary radiation exposure. This is just a precaution to minimize exposure to sensitive areas like the reproductive organs.

WHEN TO TALK TO YOUR DOCTOR?

If your doctor suggests an X-ray, it's important to discuss any concerns or ask questions, especially if you're pregnant or have had many X-rays in the past. Your doctor will ensure that X-rays are only used when absolutely necessary and that your safety is always the priority.

What is a Digital X-ray?

A **Digital X-ray** is a modern type of X-ray that takes pictures of the inside of your body using digital technology. It's similar to a traditional X-ray but with some updated features that make it faster and easier.

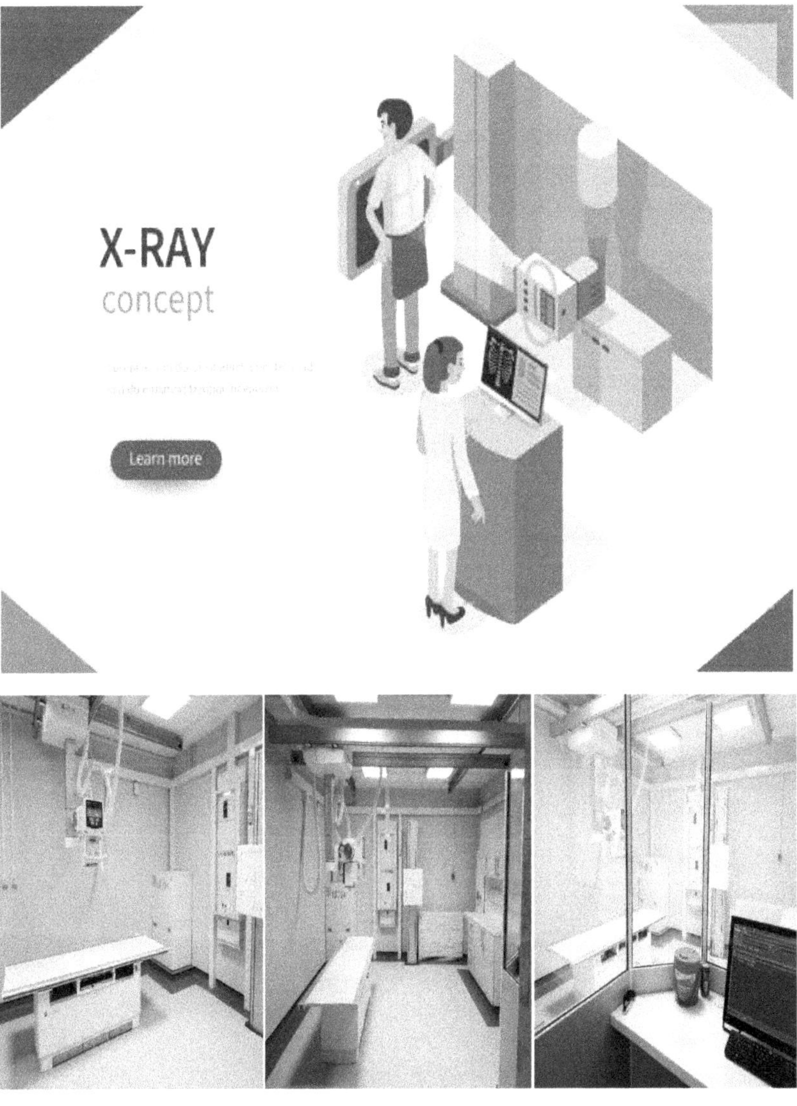

How Does It Work?

1. **X-ray Machine**: The machine sends out invisible X-rays that pass through your body.
2. **Digital Sensor**: Instead of using film like older X-rays, a digital sensor captures the X-rays. This sensor is more like a computer screen and quickly turns the X-rays into a digital image.
3. **Computer Screen**: The digital image appears on a computer screen almost instantly, allowing doctors to see and examine it right away.

What Are the Benefits?

- **Faster Results**: You get your X-ray images right away on a computer screen, so doctors can quickly review them.
- **Better Images**: Digital X-rays often provide clearer and more detailed images than traditional X-rays.
- **Less Radiation**: Digital X-rays use less radiation compared to older X-ray methods, making them safer.
- **Easy Storage**: Digital images are stored on a computer, making them easier to keep and share with other doctors if needed.

Is It Safe?

Yes, digital X-rays are safe. They use very low levels of radiation, and the benefits of getting clear, quick images generally outweigh the risks.

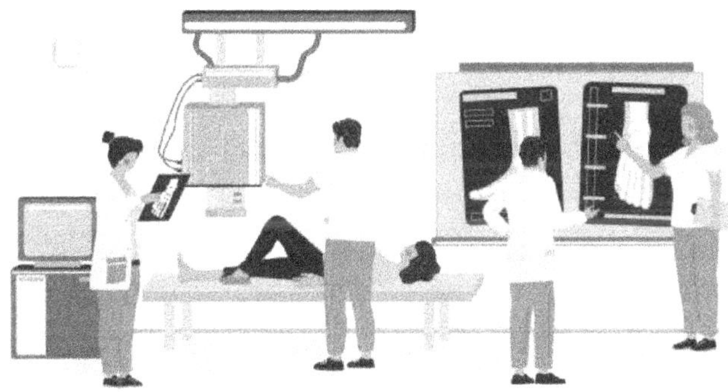

What is Fluoroscopy?

Fluoroscopy is a type of medical imaging that lets doctors see real-time, moving images of the inside of your body. It's like a live video of your organs and bones, allowing doctors to observe them in action.

How Does It Work?

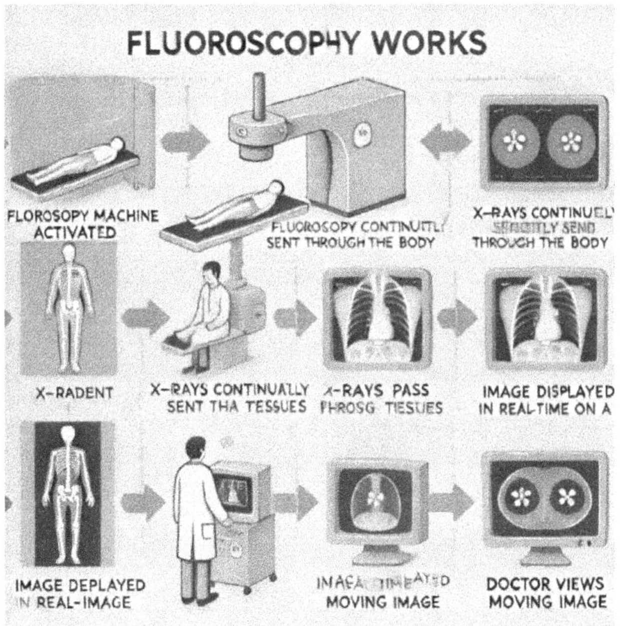

1. **X-ray Machine**: A special X-ray machine sends out a continuous beam of X-rays.
2. **Fluoroscope**: Instead of just taking a single picture, the X-rays create a live video feed that is captured by a device called a fluoroscope.
3. **Computer Screen**: The live images appear on a monitor, so doctors can see how things like your digestive system or heart are working in real-time.

What Are the Benefits?

- **Real-Time Viewing**: Doctors can watch how your organs and systems function while you move or swallow, which helps them diagnose problems more accurately.
- **Guided Procedures**: Fluoroscopy is often used to guide certain procedures, like inserting a catheter or checking the placement of medical devices.
- **Detailed Assessment**: It provides a detailed view of dynamic processes, like how well a heart valve is working or how food moves through the digestive tract.

What Happens During Fluoroscopy?

1. **Preparation**: You may need to lie down or sit in a specific position depending on what part of your body is being examined.
2. **Contrast Material**: Sometimes, you might be asked to drink or receive an injection of a special contrast material (like a dye) that helps certain parts of your body show up more clearly on the images.

3. **Live Images**: The fluoroscope will take continuous X-ray images, showing the real-time movement of the area being examined.
4. **Monitoring**: The doctor watches the images on a screen and may ask you to perform certain actions, like swallowing or moving a limb, to see how your body responds.

Is It Safe?

Fluoroscopy uses X-rays, so there is some exposure to radiation. However, the amount is usually low, and the benefits of getting detailed, real-time images often outweigh the risks. Doctors take precautions to minimize radiation exposure

WHAT IS A MAMMOGRAM?

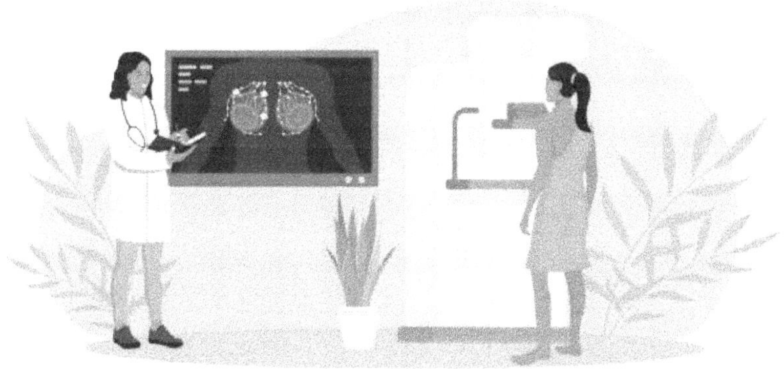

A **mammogram** is a low-dose X-ray used to take images of the breasts.

It helps doctors detect **breast cancer** and other breast abnormalities at an early stage, even before they can be felt as a lump.

Mammograms are important because they can find cancer early when it's easier to treat, potentially saving lives.

Mammography is commonly used in **breast cancer screening programs** and is a routine test recommended for most women, particularly those over 40, or younger women with a family history of breast cancer.

How does Mammography work?

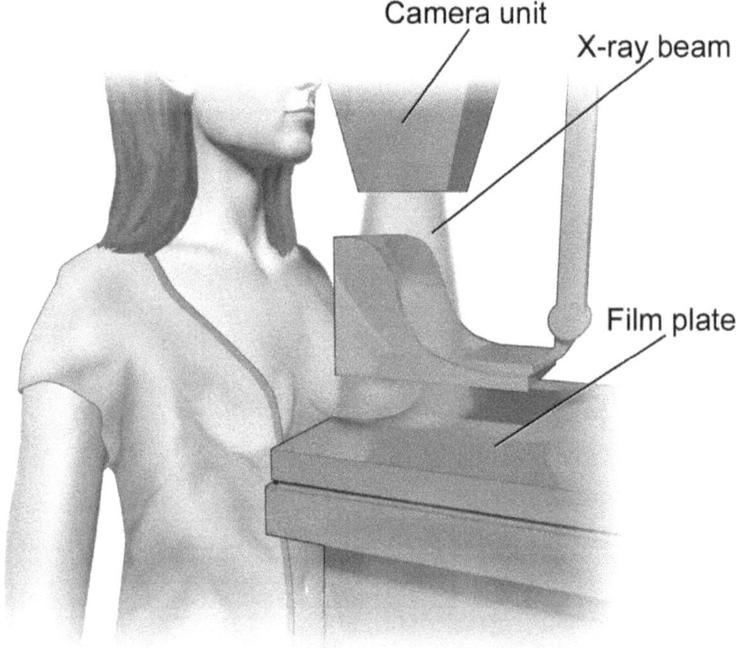

Mammogram

The process of getting a mammogram is straightforward but can cause mild discomfort for a short time. Here's a breakdown of how it works:

- **Preparation**: You will be asked to undress from the waist up and wear a gown. Before the procedure, you should avoid wearing deodorant, powders, or lotions under your arms or on your breasts because they might show up on the X-ray images and affect the results.

- **Positioning**: You'll stand in front of a special X-ray machine. The radiology technologist will help position your breast on a flat plate (detector) of the machine.
- **Compression**: A second plate is gently lowered onto your breast to flatten it. This part of the process might feel uncomfortable or cause slight pressure, but it's necessary. Flattening the breast spreads the tissue, which allows for clearer images and reduces the amount of X-ray energy needed.
- **Taking the X-ray**: Once your breast is compressed, the machine takes an X-ray. Usually, two pictures are taken of each breast: one from the top and one from the side. In some cases, additional images may be needed, depending on the size or density of your breasts.
- **Duration**: The entire mammogram procedure typically takes about 15-20 minutes. The compression itself only lasts a few seconds for each picture.

Why is a Mammogram Done? (Indications)

Mammograms are used for two main reasons:

1. **Screening Mammogram**

   A screening mammogram is done on women who have no symptoms of breast cancer. It's a routine test meant to catch early signs of cancer. Here's why it's important:

   - **Early detection**: Breast cancer can develop without noticeable symptoms. Mammograms can find lumps or other signs of cancer **years before** they can be felt. Detecting cancer early increases the chances of successful treatment.

- **Regular screening**: Women over the age of 40 (or sometimes younger with a family history) are often advised to have a mammogram every **1-2 years**. Your doctor may recommend more frequent tests based on individual risk factors, such as family history or genetic mutations like BRCA1/BRCA2.

2. **Diagnostic Mammogram**

   A diagnostic mammogram is done when a woman has symptoms such as:

   - A lump or thickening in the breast
   - Breast pain that doesn't go away
   - Unexplained changes in the size or shape of the breast
   - Nipple discharge
   - Skin changes (such as redness or dimpling)

This type of mammogram may involve more images than a screening mammogram. It helps the doctor get a closer look at any areas of concern and guide further tests, such as a **biopsy**.

Benefits of Mammography

- **Saves lives**: By detecting cancer early, mammograms help reduce the number of deaths from breast cancer, especially in women over 50.

- **Non-invasive**: A mammogram is a simple, non-surgical procedure that provides valuable information without the need for a biopsy or surgery.
- **Helps identify other issues**: In addition to cancer, mammograms can detect other problems, like **benign cysts**, **calcifications**, or **fibrocystic changes**, which may require monitoring or treatment.

Limitations and Considerations

While mammography is an excellent tool, it has some limitations:

- **False positives**: Sometimes, a mammogram can suggest something is wrong when there isn't. This can lead to additional testing and anxiety.
- **False negatives**: In rare cases, a mammogram might miss a cancer, especially in women with **dense breast tissue**, which can make it harder to see small tumors.
- **Radiation exposure**: Mammograms use a very low dose of radiation. The amount is safe, but some people worry about repeated exposure over time. However, the benefits of early detection usually outweigh the risks.

What Happens After a Mammogram?

- **Results**: The images are reviewed by a Radiologist (a doctor who specializes in interpreting medical images). If the results are normal, you continue with your regular screenings. If anything suspicious is found, you may be asked to come back for more tests, such as additional mammograms, an ultrasound, or a biopsy to get a clearer picture.

- **Follow-up**: Regular follow-up mammograms help doctors track any changes in the breast over time, which can be important for early detection.

Mammograms are a powerful tool in the fight against breast cancer. While the idea of getting a mammogram can be uncomfortable or even a little frightening, the procedure is quick and the benefits, especially in terms of early detection, are life-saving.

Before knowing more about Computerised tomography (CT),

Let's learn difference between **X-ray** and **CT scan.,**

1. **X-ray:**
   - **What it is**: An X-ray is like taking a single picture of the inside of your body. It's mainly used to look at bones and can also check for issues in the chest or teeth.
   - **How it works**: A small amount of radiation passes through your body and creates an image on a film or screen.
2. **CT Scan:**
   - **What it is**: A CT scan (Computed Tomography scan) is like taking **many X-ray pictures** from different angles, then using a computer to combine them into a detailed 3D image of the inside of your body.
   - **How it works**: The CT scanner takes multiple X-rays as it spins around your body. The images are then pieced together to provide a clearer and more detailed picture.

- **Best for**: CT scans are better for seeing **soft tissues**, **organs**, **blood vessels**, and **more complex injuries**. It helps in detecting things like tumors, internal bleeding, or issues in the brain.
- **Example**: If you've had a head injury, a CT scan can show if there's any bleeding or damage inside the brain.

In Summary:

- **X-ray** = single image, mostly for bones.
- **CT scan** = many images combined into 3D, for more detailed views of organs and tissues.

CHAPTER 6

"A CLEAR LOOK INSIDE: EXPLAINING CT SCANS FOR EVERYONE"

A **CT scan** (or **CAT scan**) stands for **Computed Tomography scan**. It's a special kind of X-ray that lets doctors see detailed pictures of the inside of your body. It's commonly used to look at bones, muscles, organs, and blood vessels.

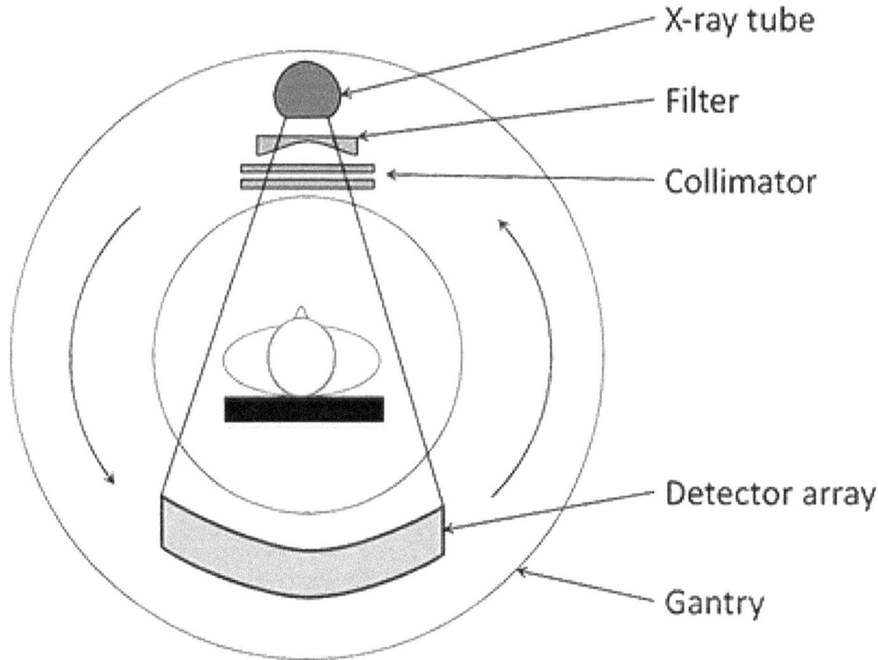

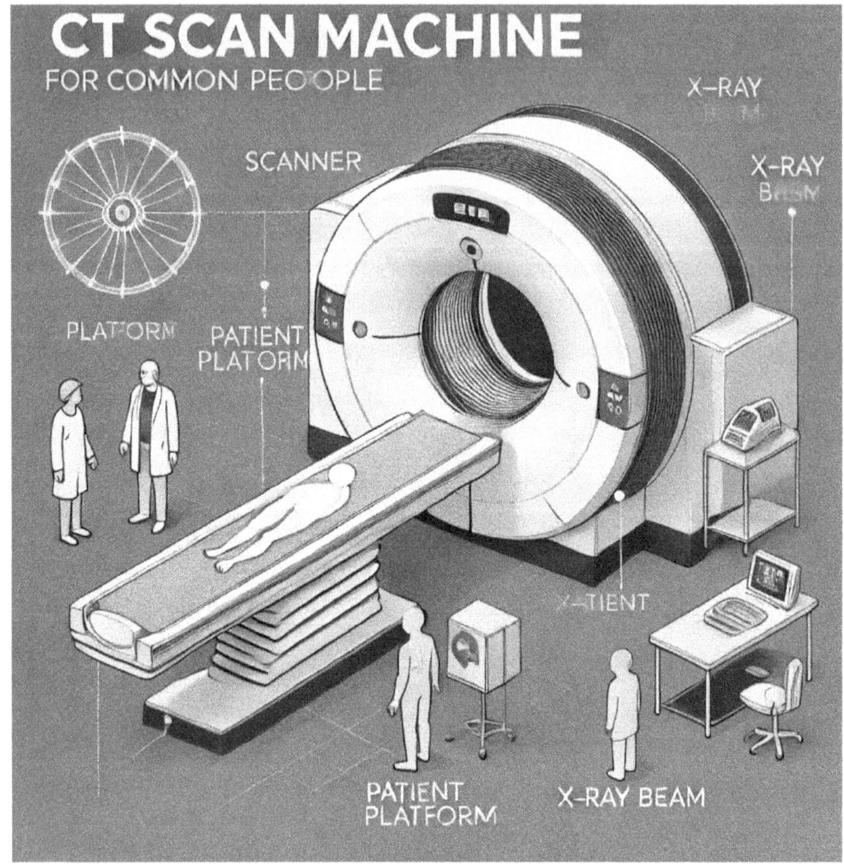

When Do You Need a CT Scan?

Doctors may ask for a CT scan if:

- You've been in an accident, and they need to check for internal injuries or broken bones.
- They need to look for tumors or growths.
- They need to examine your blood vessels or check for signs of a stroke.
- They want to see how well a treatment, like cancer therapy, is working.

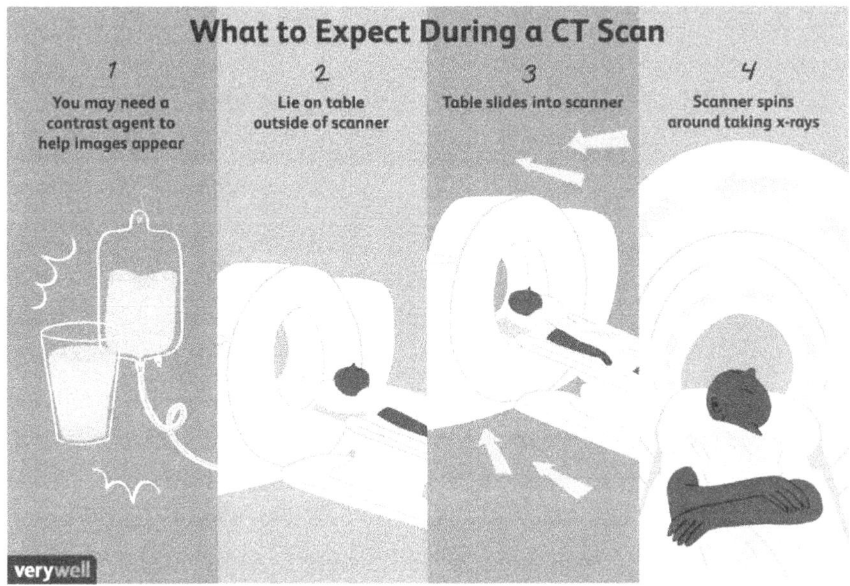

Radiation Safety Measures for a CT Scan

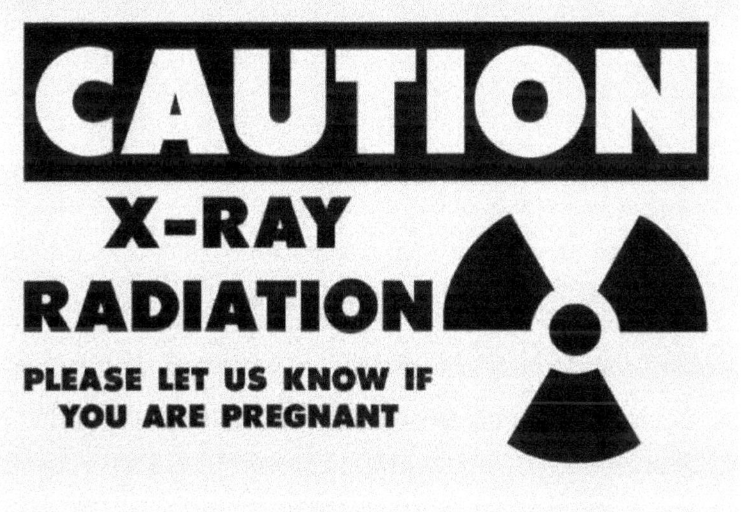

Understand the Importance of Safety: CT scans use a small amount of radiation to create detailed images of your body. While the amount of radiation is carefully controlled

and generally safe, certain steps can reduce unnecessary exposure.

Before the CT Scan

1. **Inform Your Doctor**
    - **Let your doctor know if:**
    - **You are pregnant or think you might be. (Radiation can harm an unborn baby.)**
    - **You have had multiple scans recently.**
    - **Your doctor may suggest an alternative test (like an ultrasound or MRI) if necessary.**
2. **Ask About the Scan**
    - **Ask your doctor why the scan is needed and how it will help your diagnosis.**
    - **Confirm that the scan is absolutely necessary.**
3. **Provide a Full Medical History**
    - **Share your medical history, including any conditions like kidney problems, allergies to contrast dye, or previous exposure to radiation.**
4. **Choose Accredited Centers**
    - **Ensure the scan is performed at a facility with proper accreditation and trained technicians who follow radiation safety protocols.**

During the CT Scan

1. **Use of Lead Shields**
   - **In some cases, the technician may use lead aprons or shields to protect parts of your body that don't need to be scanned (e.g., thyroid gland, reproductive organs).**
2. **Minimizing Scan Area**
   - **The technician will focus the radiation only on the specific area being examined to avoid unnecessary exposure to the rest of your body.**
3. **Low-Dose Settings**
   - **Modern CT scanners often use low-dose settings to reduce radiation exposure while still getting clear images.**
4. **Follow Instructions**
   - **Stay still and follow the technician's instructions carefully. The scan is quick, and staying still prevents the need for repeated scans.**

Additional Tips

- **If Contrast Dye Is Used:**
  - **The contrast dye highlights certain areas in your body for a clearer scan. It does not increase radiation exposure.**
  - **Let the doctor know if you've had reactions to contrast dye in the past.**

- **For Children:**
    - **If the scan is for a child, ensure the medical team uses pediatric settings to limit radiation exposure.**

After the CT Scan

- **There is no residual radiation in your body after a CT scan.**
- **Drink plenty of water if contrast dye was used to help flush it from your system.**

Is It Safe?

Yes, a CT scan is generally safe. It uses X-rays, so you'll be exposed to a small amount of radiation, but doctors make sure to keep the amount as low as possible. The benefits of getting a clear image far outweigh the risks.

How Long Does It Take?

The actual CT scan usually only takes **10 to 30 minutes**. Most of the time is spent getting you ready for the scan and positioning you correctly on the table. After the scan, you can usually go home right away unless your doctor needs to talk to you about the results.

Does It Hurt?

No, the CT scan itself doesn't hurt. You just have to stay still while the machine does its work. If you feel uncomfortable lying on the table, let the technician know, and they may be able to help you adjust.

What If I Feel Nervous?

Some people feel nervous or claustrophobic about being inside the machine. If you’re worried, you can talk to your doctor before the scan. The machine is open at both ends, and you can see out, so it’s not like being in a tunnel. The scan is quick, and most people find it’s easier than they expected.

Conclusion

A CT scan is a useful tool that helps doctors see inside your body in more detail than a regular X-ray.

It’s a safe and painless procedure that can help diagnose a wide range of medical conditions.

If you ever need a CT scan, now you know what to expect, and you can feel more comfortable about the process.

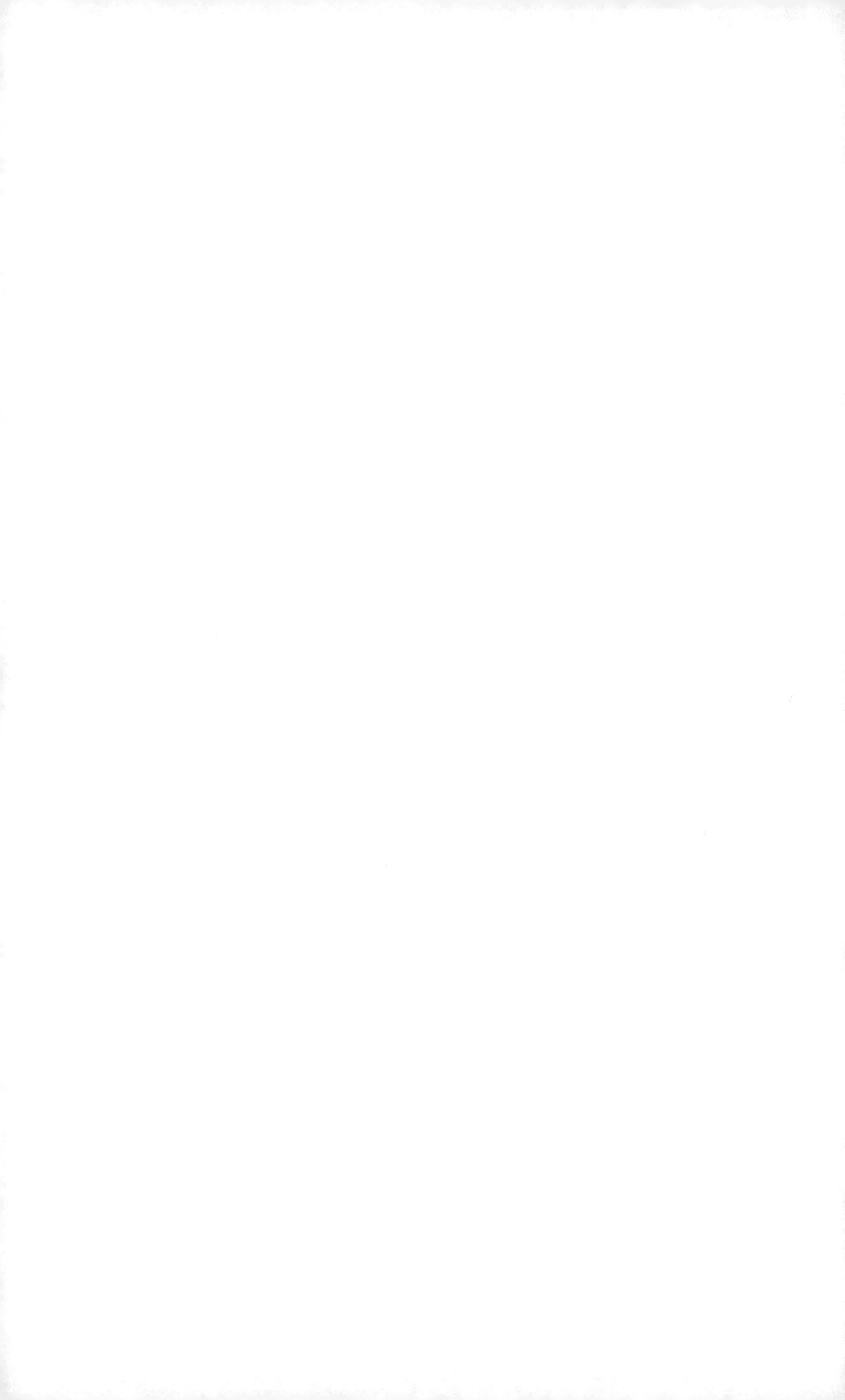

CHAPTER 7

WHAT IS SONOGRAPHY (ULTRASOUND)?

Sonography, often called **ultrasound**, is a medical test that uses **sound waves** to create pictures of the inside of your body.

Unlike X-rays, which use radiation, ultrasound uses sound waves to look inside you.

How Does Sonography Work?

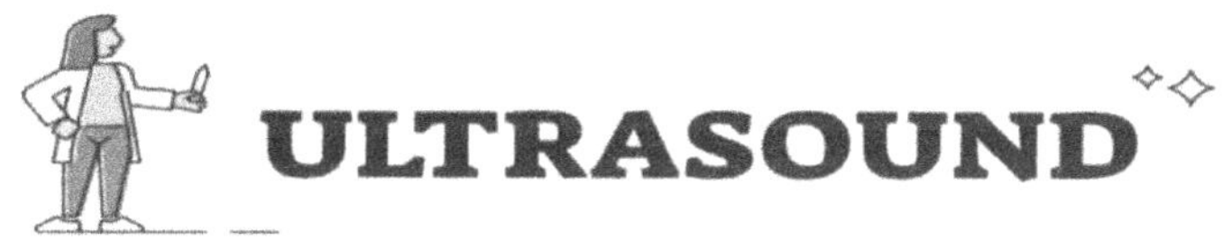

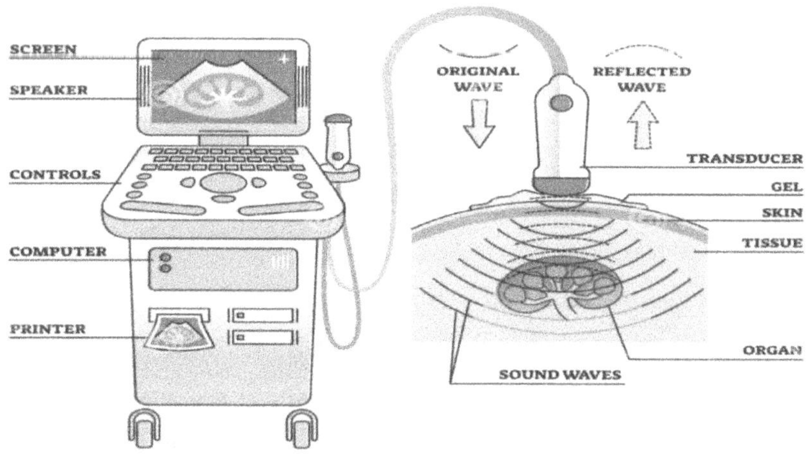

Here's how it works:

1. **Sound Waves**: An ultrasound machine sends out high-frequency sound waves that travel through your body.
2. **Echoes**: These sound waves bounce off different tissues and organs. For example, sound waves bounce back differently from bones compared to soft tissues.
3. **Images**: The machine picks up these echoes and uses them to create real-time images on a screen. These images help doctors see what's happening inside your body.

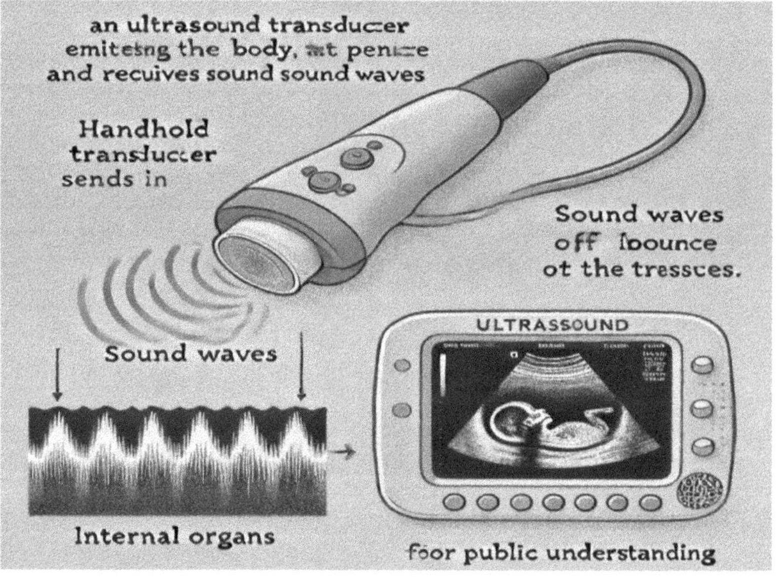

What is Sonography Used For?

Sonography can be used for many things, such as:

- **Checking Baby's Health**: It's commonly used during pregnancy to see how the baby is growing and to check the baby's health.

- **Examining Organs**: It helps doctors look at organs like the liver, kidneys, and heart to find any issues.
- **Diagnosing Problems**: It can help find problems like tumors, cysts, or infections in various parts of the body.
- **Guiding Procedures**: Sometimes, ultrasound is used to guide doctors during certain medical procedures.

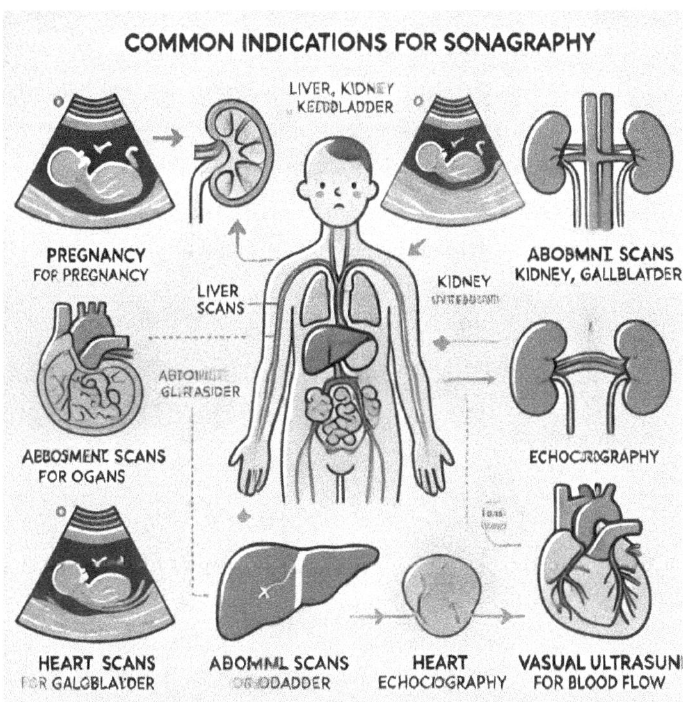

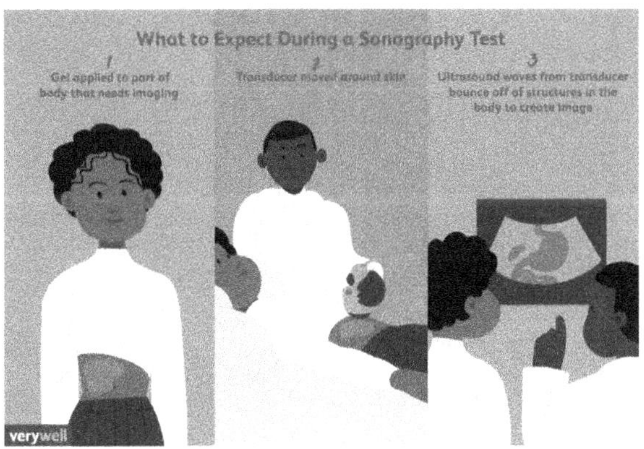

What To Expect From Your Ultrasound Exam

Diagnostic medical sonography (ultrasound) turns sound waves into images used to diagnose disease and injury, monitor health and guide medical treatment. If a healthcare professional has ordered an ultrasound examination for you, here's what you need to know!

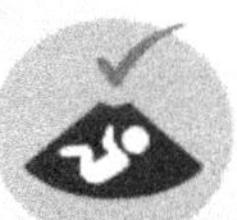

Ultrasound is safe for patients and fetuses when it's used by a qualified, credentialed sonographer.
Ask your sonographer about their training and credentials!

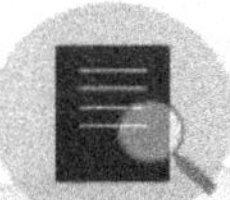

Follow all pre-appointment instructions – e.g., whether to eat or drink, take medications or empty your bladder – for the most complete and thorough exam

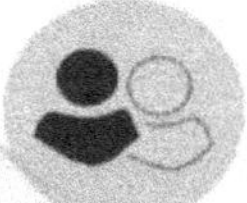

You may or may not be allowed to bring someone with you into the scan room so the sonographer can focus on the exam

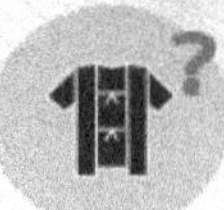

This is a medical exam. Your sonographer may ask you about your symptoms and health history, and to put on a gown or to adjust/remove clothing

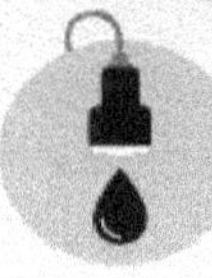

Gel or lotion will be applied to maintain contact between the probe and your skin to make imaging possible

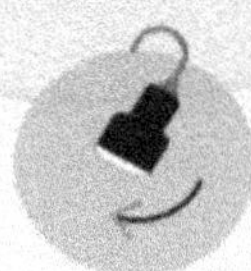

A probe will be placed on or in the area to be examined and adjusted to capture images

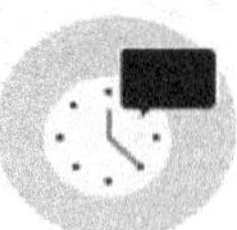

Scans can take 25 minutes or up to 2 hours – ask ahead

The sonographer will prepare a summary (including details about your history, symptoms and findings) which is sent, along with the images, to a physician for interpretation

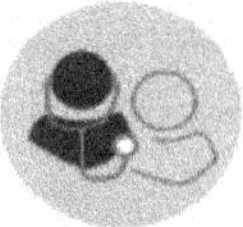

Only your physician can give you the results of your ultrasound and what it means for your health – the sonographer's job is to investigate and capture images so doctors can make sound decisions

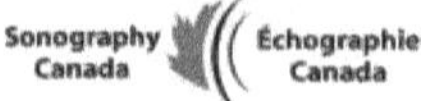

sonographycanada.ca

#SonographersSaveLives
#FrontlineHeroesEveryDay

How to Prepare for Sonography:

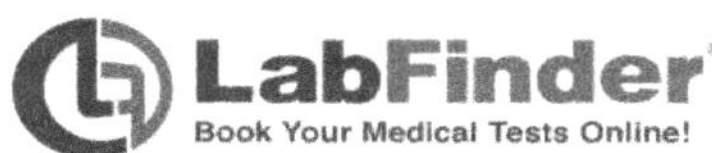

Preparation Guidelines for Ultrasounds

Breast, Carotid and Thyroid ultrasounds do not require any preparation.

Abdominal/Gall Bladder Ultrasound Preparation Instructions:

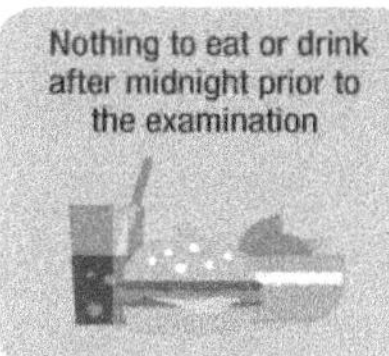

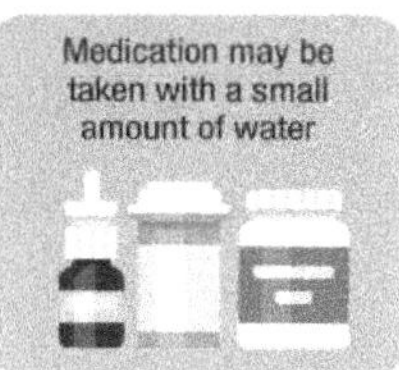

Renal, Obstetrical & Pelvic Ultrasound Preparation Instructions:

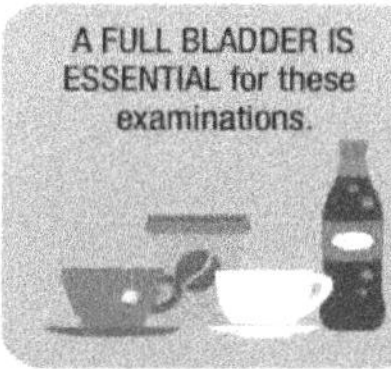

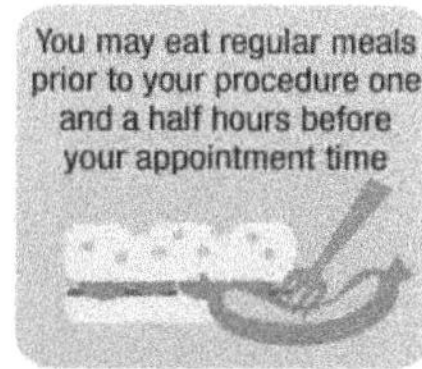

*Obstetrical and Pelvic Ultrasounds - drink 32 oz. of water (4 large glasses).
*Renal Ultrasound - drink 20 oz. of water prior to test.

- Try to keep your bladder full for the test
- DO NOT go to the washroom until after your examination
- Allow 30 minutes for the exam

If the instructions are not followed, another appointment will have to be made.

Note: Women should always inform their doctor and Radiology Center if they are, or think they might be pregnant.

Should you have any further concerns and inquiries, please contact your doctor or radiology center.

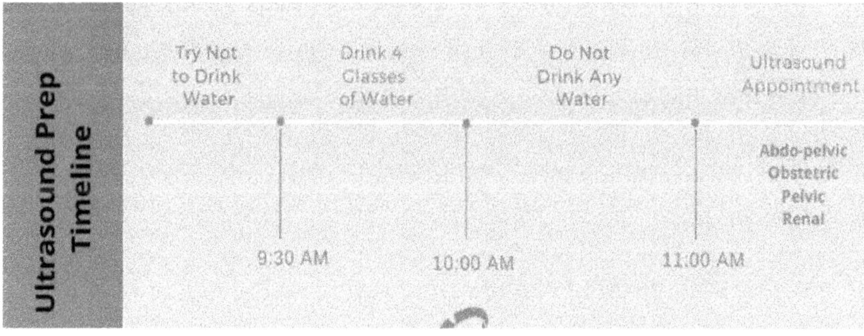

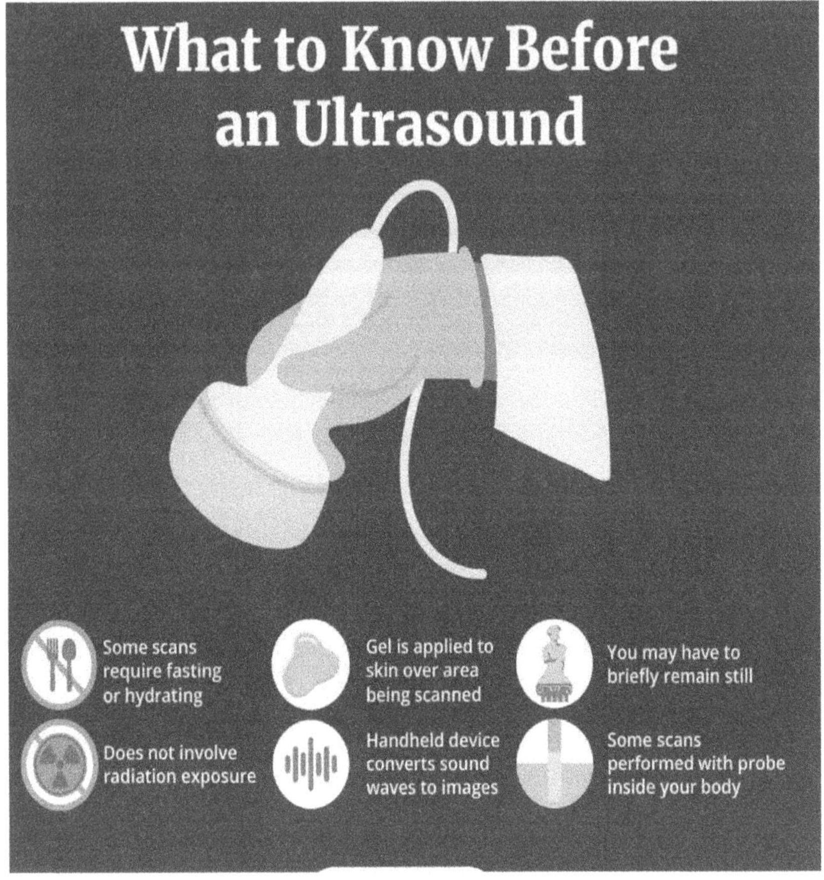

1. **Drink Water (for some tests):**

   - For an ultrasound of the **pelvis** or during **pregnancy**, you might be asked to drink several glasses of water before the test and **not go to the bathroom**. A full bladder helps the technician get clearer images.

   - **Tip**: Make sure you don't empty your bladder until after the scan.

2. **Fasting (for some tests):**

   - If you're having an ultrasound of the **abdomen** (like the liver, gallbladder, or pancreas), you may need to **avoid**

eating or drinking for 8-12 hours before the test. This is because food and liquids in your stomach can make it harder to see certain organs clearly.

3. **Comfortable Clothing:**
   - Wear **loose, comfortable clothing**. You might be asked to lift your shirt or lower your waistband for the scan, depending on the area being examined.
   - For some types of ultrasound, you may need to wear a **hospital gown**.
4. **No Special Preparation (for some tests):**
   - For ultrasounds of the **heart** (echocardiogram), **thyroid**, or other parts of the body, there's usually **no special preparation** required. You can eat and drink as usual.

During the Scan:

- **Gel**: The technician will apply a special **gel** on your skin to help the ultrasound device move smoothly and transmit sound waves. The gel might feel a little cool but is harmless.
- **Transducer**: A small device called a **transducer** will be moved over the area being checked. It sends sound waves into your body and creates the images.
- **Painless**: The process is painless and takes about **15-30 minutes**, depending on the area being scanned.
- **Stay Still**: You may be asked to **hold your breath** or stay still for a few seconds to get clearer images.

After the Scan:

- You can **go to the bathroom** and **resume normal activities** right away. There are no side effects from the scan, and the gel can easily be wiped off.

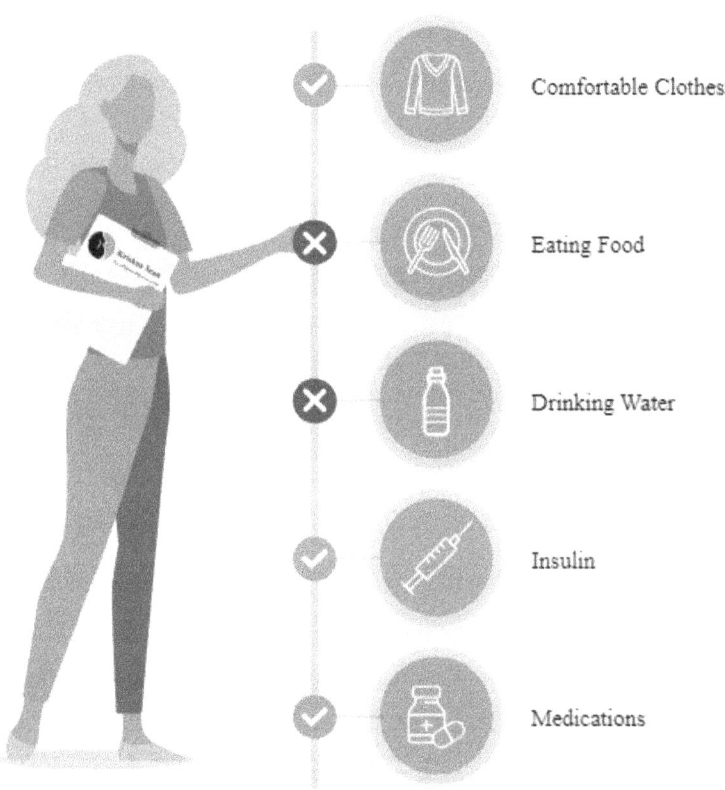

LET'S BREAK DOWN SOME OF THESE COMMON MYTHS AND REVEAL THE TRUTH BEHIND THEM:

1. **Myth: Ultrasound uses radiation**
    - **Fact**: Unlike X-rays and CT scans, ultrasound imaging **does not use radiation**. Instead, it employs

high-frequency sound waves to create images of the body's internal structures. This makes it a safe option, especially for sensitive populations like pregnant women and infants.

2. **Myth: Ultrasounds are only for pregnancy**
   - **Fact**: While ultrasounds are famously used for monitoring pregnancies, they are used for **a wide range of medical applications**. These include:
     - Examining the heart (Echocardiograms)
     - Checking organs like the liver, kidneys, and bladder
     - Diagnosing conditions like gallstones, tumors, and blood vessel blockages
3. **Myth: Ultrasounds always provide a clear diagnosis**
   - **Fact**: Ultrasound is a valuable diagnostic tool, but it has **limitations**. The clarity of images depends on factors like the patient's body size, the location of the organ, or the presence of gas (such as in the intestines), which can obstruct sound waves. Sometimes, additional imaging techniques like CT or MRI are needed for more detailed results.
4. **Myth: Sonography is painful**
   - **Fact**: **Sonography is generally painless**. Most procedures involve placing a small probe (transducer) on the skin after applying a gel that helps transmit sound waves. The process is non-invasive and causes little to no discomfort. In some cases,a transvaginal or transrectal ultrasound may be used, but even then, discomfort is usually minimal.

5. **Myth: Ultrasound can harm the baby during pregnancy**
   - **Fact**: Ultrasound imaging is **considered very safe for both mother and baby**. It has been used for decades in prenatal care with no evidence of harm. It uses sound waves rather than radiation, making it a safer option for monitoring fetal development compared to other imaging methods.
6. **Myth: 3D/4D ultrasounds are only for fun or entertainment**
   - **Fact**: While **3D and 4D ultrasounds** are often used to create "keepsake" images and videos of babies in the womb, they also have important **medical uses**. For instance, they can provide detailed images of the baby's anatomy, helping to diagnose conditions like cleft lip, spinal issues, or other abnormalities. However, non-medical use of these ultrasounds is discouraged unless necessary.
7. **Myth: Ultrasound can detect everything**
   - **Fact**: While ultrasounds are powerful diagnostic tools, they **cannot detect all medical conditions**. For example, ultrasounds are not as effective for imaging bones or organs that are surrounded by air, such as the lungs. In such cases, other imaging methods like X-ray, CT or MRIs are preferred.
8. **Myth: Ultrasound can predict the exact due date**
   - **Fact**: While ultrasounds can provide an **estimated due date**, they are not 100% accurate. The most accurate time for predicting the due date is during

the first trimester. Later in pregnancy, factors like baby's growth rate or movement can affect the estimated due date, making it less precise.

9. **Myth: All ultrasounds are the same**

   - **Fact**: There are **different types of ultrasounds**, each with specific uses:

     - **2D Ultrasound**: The most common type, which produces flat, two-dimensional images.
     - **3D Ultrasound**: Provides three-dimensional, more life like images.
     - **4D Ultrasound**: Adds the dimension of movement, creating real-time video images.
     - **Doppler Ultrasound**: Measures blood flow and is often used to assess heart and blood vessel conditions.

Conclusion:

Ultrasound (sonography) is a versatile and safe imaging technique with various uses beyond pregnancy. While myths and misconceptions persist, understanding the facts can help patients feel more comfortable and informed about the procedure.

MYTHS AND FACTS ABOUT PREGNANCY SCANS

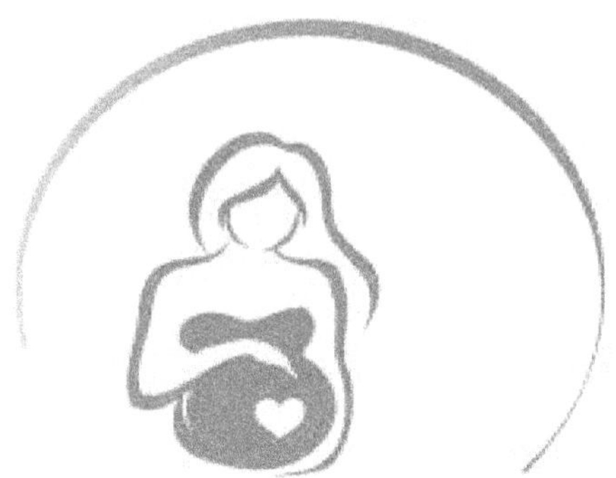

Myth 1: Pregnancy scans are harmful to the baby.

- Fact: Ultrasound scans are considered very safe for both the mother and the baby. They use sound waves rather than radiation, which eliminates the risk associated with X-rays. Extensive research and years of use have shown no harmful effects from routine ultrasounds.

Myth 2: You only need a scan if there's a problem.

- Fact: Routine pregnancy scans are used to monitor the health and development of the baby and to check for any potential issues early on. They provide important information about the baby's growth, the position of the placenta, and the amount of amniotic fluid.

Myth 3: Ultrasound can determine the exact birth date.

- Fact: While ultrasounds can provide an estimated due date, it is not always precise. Due dates can change based on the baby's growth and other factors. The most accurate estimates are given early in pregnancy when the baby is still small and developing at a predictable rate.

Myth 4: 3D and 4D ultrasounds are necessary for medical purposes.

- Fact: 3D and 4D ultrasounds are often used for creating detailed images and videos of the baby, which can be memorable for parents. However, 2D ultrasounds are generally sufficient for medical evaluations and monitoring the baby's health and development.

Myth 5: You should have as many ultrasounds as possible to ensure the baby's health.

- Fact: While ultrasounds are useful, they should be done only as necessary based on medical advice. Routine scans are usually scheduled at specific times during pregnancy. Excessive or unnecessary scans are not recommended and should be avoided unless there is a medical reason.

Myth 6: Ultrasound scans can predict the baby's future health.

- Fact: Ultrasounds can provide valuable information about the baby's current health and development, but they cannot predict future health conditions. Some conditions may not be detectable through ultrasound, and ongoing care and assessments are important.

Myth 7: Ultrasound can reveal the baby's personality or characteristics.

- Fact: While ultrasounds can show physical features and general anatomy, they cannot determine personality traits or other characteristics. They are used to assess physical development and health.

Myth 8: If a scan shows no issues, you don't need to worry about the baby's health.

- Fact: While a normal scan is reassuring, it's important to continue regular prenatal care. Ultrasounds are one part of monitoring pregnancy, and ongoing care includes other assessments and evaluations to ensure both mother and baby remain healthy.

Myth 9: All ultrasound machines are the same.

- Fact: There are different types of ultrasound machines with varying levels of detail and clarity. Advanced machines may provide more detailed images, but even basic machines can offer crucial information for monitoring the pregnancy

Myth 10: You can always see the baby's gender clearly.

- Fact: Determining the baby's gender depends on factors such as the baby's position and the clarity of the image. Sometimes, it may be difficult to see clearly, especially in early scans or if the baby is not positioned in an optimal way.

Indications for Transvaginal Sonography.

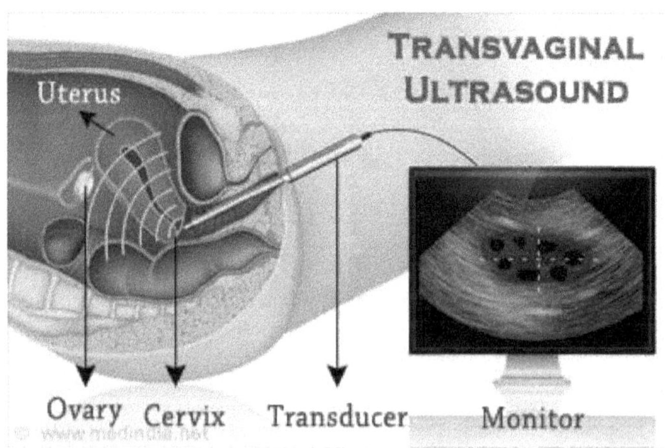

1. **Early Pregnancy Assessment**:
    - **Confirming Pregnancy**: To verify an early pregnancy when it's too early to see with a standard abdominal ultrasound.
    - **Determining Gestational Age**: To measure the embryo or fetus and estimate the due date more accurately.
    - **Checking for Ectopic Pregnancy**: To ensure the pregnancy is developing within the uterus and not in an abnormal location, such as the fallopian tubes.
2. **Evaluating Pelvic Pain**:
    - **Identifying Causes of Pain**: To help diagnose the cause of pelvic pain or discomfort, such as ovarian cysts, endometriosis, or pelvic inflammatory disease.
3. **Assessing Uterine and Ovarian Health**:
    - **Checking Uterine Abnormalities**: To evaluate conditions like fibroids, polyps, or uterine malformations.
    - **Examining Ovarian Masses**: To investigate the presence of ovarian cysts, tumors, or other abnormalities.
4. **Investigating Abnormal Bleeding**:
    - **Diagnosing Abnormal Bleeding**: To understand the cause of irregular bleeding or spotting, and to assess conditions such as abnormal endometrial thickening or cancer.
5. **Monitoring Fertility Treatments**:
    - **Assessing Follicle Development**: To monitor the growth of ovarian follicles during fertility treatments and assist in timing ovulation or egg retrieval.

6. **Guiding Procedures**:
   - **Performing Biopsies**: To guide biopsies or other procedures on pelvic organs.
   - **Assisting with Intrauterine Device (IUD) Placement**: To ensure the correct placement and positioning of an IUD.
7. **Evaluating Pelvic Organ Prolapse**:
   - **Diagnosing Prolapse**: To assess the extent of pelvic organ prolapse, where organs like the bladder or uterus may drop into the vaginal canal.
8. **Checking for Signs of Infection**:
   - **Detecting Pelvic Infections**: To find evidence of infections, such as abscesses or inflammatory conditions.
9. **Pre- and Post-Surgical Evaluation**:
   - **Assessing Post-Surgical Recovery**: To check for complications or assess healing after pelvic surgery.
10. **Screening for Certain Cancers**:
    - **Monitoring for Cancer**: In some cases, to evaluate for signs of cancers such as endometrial or ovarian cancer, especially in high-risk individuals.

Conclusion

Transvaginal sonography provides detailed images that are crucial for diagnosing and managing various gynecological and obstetric conditions.

It allows doctors to see structures in greater detail compared to external ultrasound, which can lead to more accurate diagnoses and treatment plans.

If you have any questions or need further details, feel free to ask your docotr.

ECHOCARDIOGRAPHY: A WINDOW TO THE HEART

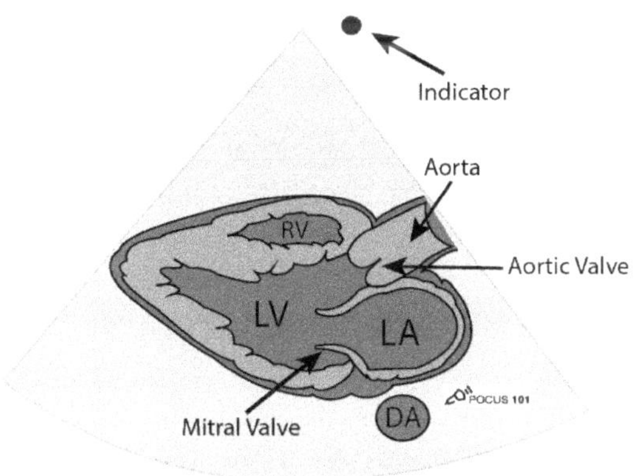

Echocardiography is like a live-action movie of your heart, created using sound waves. This non-invasive, painless test helps doctors see your heart's size, shape, and movement in real-time.

It's often used to assess how well your heart pumps blood and to detect problems with heart valves, muscles, or surrounding structures.

Why Echocardiography is Important

- **Early Detection of Heart Problems**: It can spot heart issues like weak pumping (heart failure), leaky or narrowed valves, or structural abnormalities before they cause severe symptoms.
- **Guides Treatment**: For people with heart conditions, it helps doctors decide the best treatment—whether that's medication, surgery, or lifestyle changes.

- **Monitors Progress**: For ongoing conditions, it tracks how well treatments are working.
- **Common Types of Echocardiograms**
- **Transthoracic Echocardiogram (TTE)**: The standard test where a probe is placed on the chest.
- **Transesophageal Echocardiogram (TEE)**: A probe is passed down the esophagus for clearer images, often used in more complex cases.
- **Stress Echocardiogram**: Done after exercise or medication to check how the heart handles stress.
- **Doppler Echocardiogram**: Measures blood flow to detect abnormalities like leaky valves or blockages.

Echocardiography: Your Heart's Ultrasound Camera

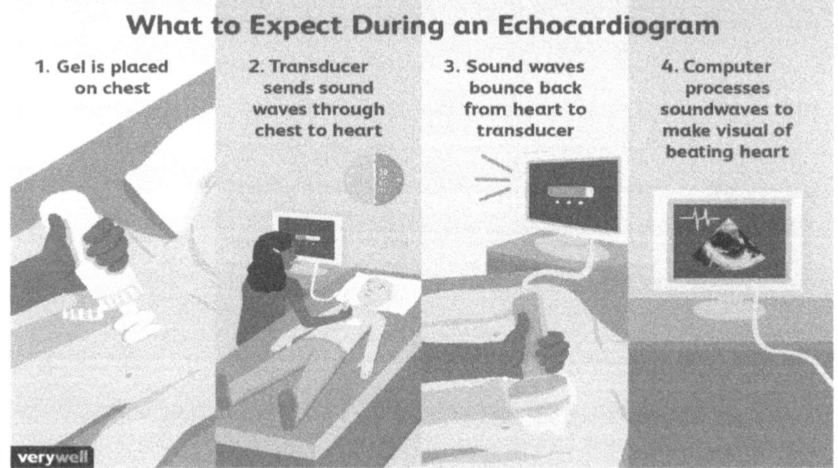

CHAPTER 8

What is an MRI?

An **MRI** (Magnetic Resonance Imaging) is a medical scan that creates detailed pictures of the inside of your body using **magnetism and radio waves**. Unlike X-rays or CT scans, an MRI **doesn't use radiation**, making it very safe.

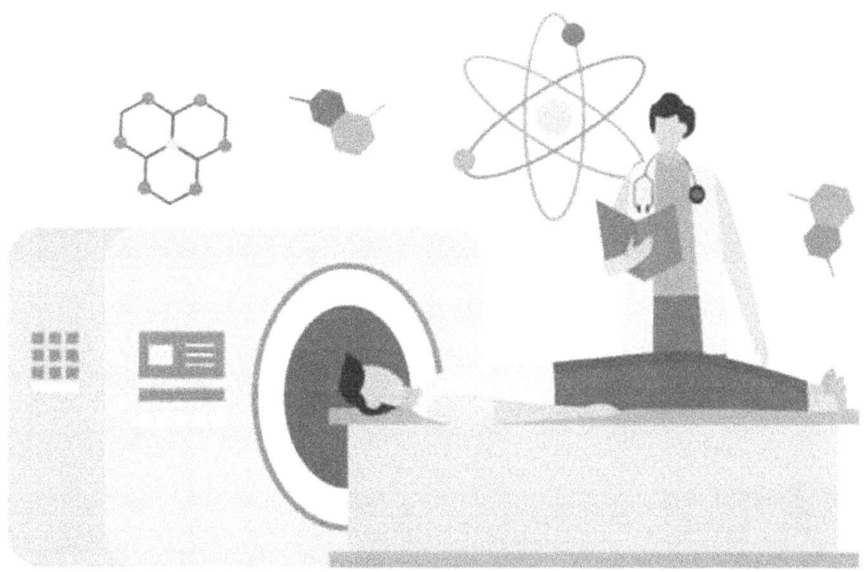

MRI

How does MRI work?

- **Big Magnet**: You lie down inside a large, tube-shaped machine that has a powerful magnet.

- **Body's Water Molecules**: The magnet interacts with the water in your body (which is everywhere in your tissues and organs).
- **Radio Waves**: The MRI machine sends radio waves into your body, which "excite" the water molecules.
- **Images Created**: When the radio waves stop, the molecules return to normal, releasing signals. The machine picks up these signals and a computer creates very detailed images of your body's insides.

MRI is especially good at imaging **soft tissues**, like your brain, muscles, and organs.

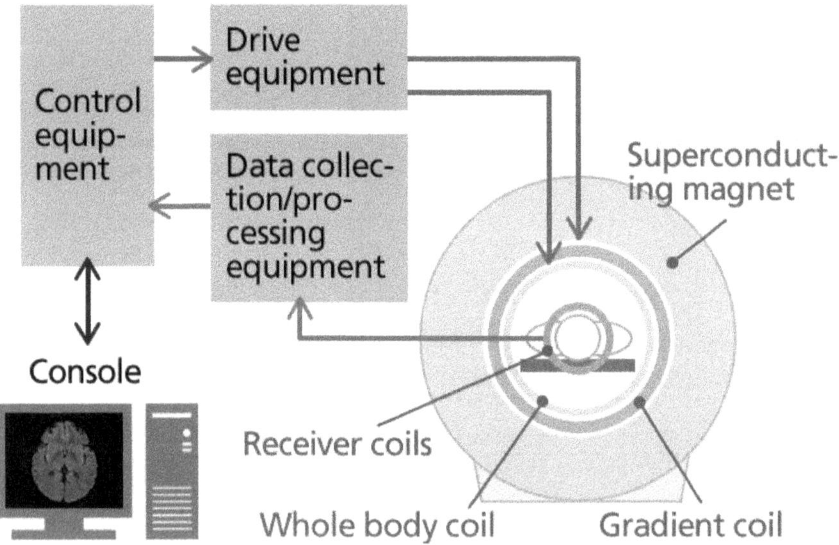

Magnetic Resonance Imaging Machine

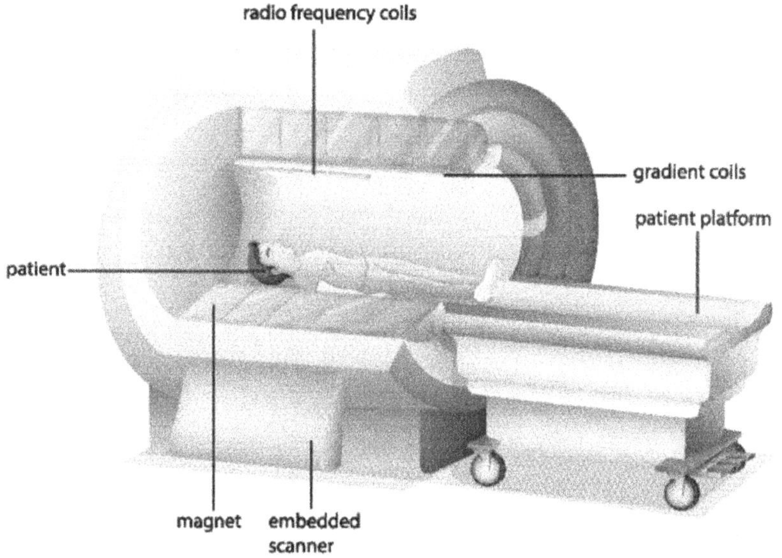

MRI examination	Indications
Brain	Ischemia, sinus thrombosis, dissection, vascular malformations, temporal epilepsy, infection, tumors, multiple sclerosis (MS), dementia, congenital abnormalities, metabolic disease, pituitary pathology, internal auditory canal pathology
Spinal cord	Pre and postoperative HNP, radiculopathy, myelopathy, MS, infection, tumors
Musculoskeletal	Joints, muscles/tendons, cartilage, infection, tumors, arthropathies
Abdomen/pelvis	Characteristic hepatic/adrenal lesions, MRCP, pancreatic pathology, intestines (appendicitis, IBD (rectal carcinoma), prostate carcinomas, cervical carcinomas, perianal fistulas, endometriosis
Cardiovascular	Ischemia, cardiomyopathies, intracardial tumors, anatomy of large vessels (including aneurysmal screening), infection/inflammation (including myocarditis), vasculitis, sinus thrombosis
Mammography	Characterization & extent of tumors
Pregnancy	Fetal anomalies

Brain MRI

A brain or head MRI shows the structures inside your head, including:

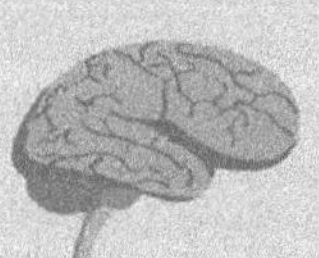

Your brain.

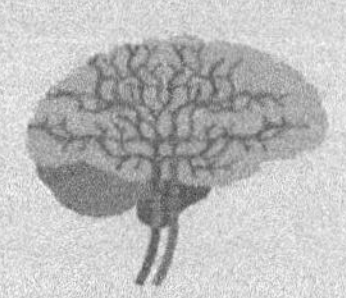

Blood vessels that connect to your brain.

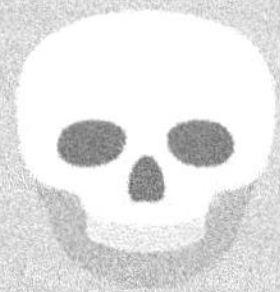

Your skull and facial bones.

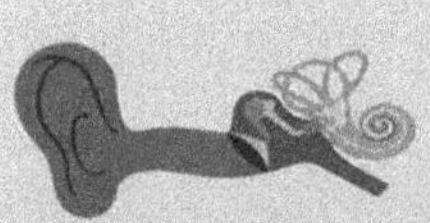

Structures in your inner ear.

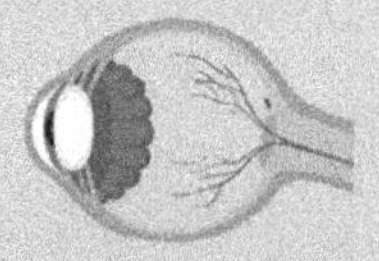

Structures in your inner eye.

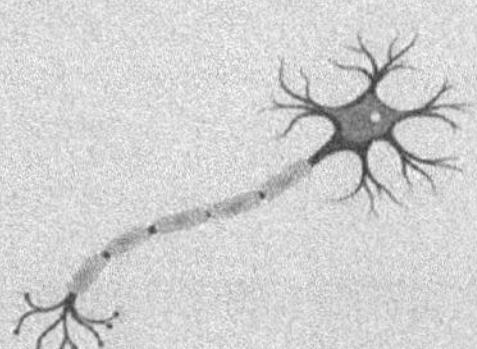

Other nerves.

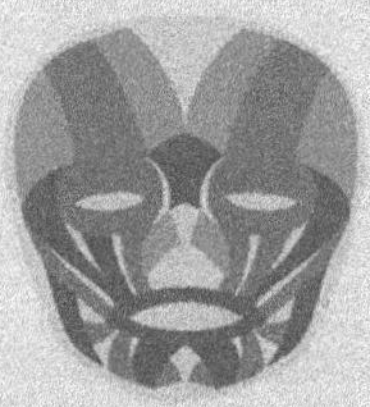

Surrounding soft tissues and skull based structures, such as fat, bones, muscle and connective tissue.

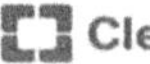

CT Scan vs. MRI: Key Differences

Aspect	CT Scan	MRI
How it works	Uses X-rays to take images.	Uses magnets and radio waves.
Best for viewing	Bones, lungs, injuries, internal bleeding.	Soft tissues like brain, muscles, organs.
Speed	Faster, takes just a few minutes.	Slower, usually takes 20-60 minutes.
Radiation	Uses radiation, like an X-ray.	No radiation, safe for repeated use.
Noise	Fairly quiet, similar to X-rays.	Loud tapping or banging sounds.
Claustrophobia	Shorter, more open machine.	Longer tube-like machine (some people feel claustrophobic).
Cost	Generally less expensive.	Generally more expensive.

When is a CT Scan Used?

- **Emergency situations: CT scans are fast, so they are often used in emergency situations like after a car accident to check for internal injuries or bleeding.**
- **Bone injuries: It's really good at showing broken bones and fractures.**
- **Chest and lungs: CT scans are helpful for looking at the lungs to check for pneumonia, lung cancer, or blood clots.**

- **Abdominal problems: It can quickly show problems in the abdomen, like appendicitis or kidney stones.**

When is an MRI Used?

- **Brain and spinal cord: MRI is the go-to test for brain problems (like strokes or tumors) and for spine issues (like herniated discs).**
- **Soft tissue injuries: It's better for seeing soft tissues like muscles, tendons, and ligaments, so it's often used for sports injuries.**
- **Organs and glands: MRI is used to look closely at organs like the liver, kidneys, and heart without radiation.**
- **Pregnancy: Since MRI doesn't use radiation, it's safer for pregnant women when imaging is needed.**

CT Scan vs. MRI: Pros and Cons

CT Scan Pros:

- **Faster: CT scans take only a few minutes, so they're great in emergencies.**
- **Better for bones: It's the best test for seeing detailed images of bones and hard tissues.**
- **Less claustrophobic: The machine is more open, making it more comfortable for people who don't like tight spaces.**

CT Scan Cons:

- **Radiation: Since it uses X-rays, there's a small amount of radiation exposure, which can be harmful if used too often.**

MRI Pros:

- **No radiation: It's safe for everyone, including pregnant women, since it doesn't use radiation.**
- **More detail: MRI is better at showing soft tissues like the brain, muscles, and organs, which helps doctors see problems more clearly.**

MRI Cons:

- **Takes longer: MRI scans usually take 20 to 60 minutes, so it's not as quick as a CT scan.**
- **Loud and confined: The MRI machine makes loud noises, and you have to lie still inside a tube, which some people find uncomfortable.**

Simple Analogy:

- **CT Scan: Imagine taking a picture of your house from different angles. A CT scan puts those pictures together to create a 3D image. It's faster but uses radiation, like a special kind of X-ray.**

- **MRI: Imagine using a super-powerful camera to see every little detail inside your house—down to the rooms and furniture. An MRI takes longer, but it shows more detail without using radiation.**

Which One is Better?

It depends on the situation:

- **If doctors need quick results (like in an emergency), or if they want to see bones or hard tissues, a CT scan is usually better.**
- **If doctors need to see soft tissues like the brain, muscles, or organs in high detail, an MRI is the better option.**

Both tests are valuable tools, and your doctor will choose the best one based on your health needs!

MRI Safety: Keeping You Safe in the Magnetic Zone

Magnetic Resonance Imaging (MRI) is a powerful tool for diagnosing health issues, but it comes with a unique safety consideration—its strong magnetic field. Think of an MRI scanner like a giant magnet that never turns off. Understanding how to stay safe during an MRI is simple when you know what to expect.

Why is MRI Safety Important?

- The MRI machine's magnetic field can attract certain metals, turning them into dangerous projectiles.

- It can interfere with some implanted medical devices like pacemakers or hearing aids.
- Knowing the rules keeps you safe while ensuring the test works properly.

How to Prepare for an MRI

Screening Questionnaire

Before your MRI, you'll fill out a questionnaire about your medical history. Be honest about any implants, surgeries, or metal in your body.

Remove All Metal Items

Leave jewelry, watches, eyeglasses, hairpins, and other metallic objects at home or in a locker. Even small metal fragments, like from old injuries, need to be checked.

Clothing

You may need to change into a hospital gown to ensure your clothing doesn't have hidden metal parts, like zippers or snaps.

What Happens During the MRI?

- **Positioning**: You'll lie on a comfortable table that slides into the MRI machine.
- **Stillness**: Staying still is crucial to get clear images.
- **Noise**: You'll hear loud knocking or buzzing sounds as the machine works, so earplugs or headphones are provided.
- **Communication**: You can talk to the technician through a microphone at any time.

Who Needs Special Attention?

- **People with Implants**: Certain devices like pacemakers, cochlear implants, or some artificial joints may not be safe for MRI. However, many modern implants are MRI-compatible. Always tell your doctor.
- **Pregnant Individuals**: MRI is generally safe during pregnancy but should be done only if absolutely necessary.
- **Metal Workers or Veterans**: If you've been exposed to metal fragments, you may need additional screening to ensure safety.

Key Takeaways for MRI Safety

1. **Be Honest**: Always share your full medical and surgical history.
2. **Metal-Free Zone**: Avoid bringing anything metallic into the MRI room.
3. **Trust the Team**: The radiology team ensures every precaution is taken for your safety.

Having an MRI?

If you can, please try and remove or don't wear:

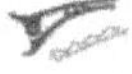 **Hair** clips & grips

 **Wigs,** hairpieces, weaves or extensions

 **Piercings,** including dermal

 **Clothing that includes metal,** e.g. bras, pants with magnets, zips or buckles

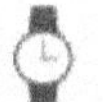 **Watches & activity trackers / rings**

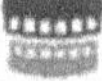 **Dentures** containing metal

 **Jewellery & glasses**

 **Facemasks** containing metal

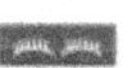 **Fake eyelashes**

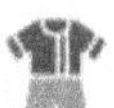 **Sport clothing** that contains silver fibres

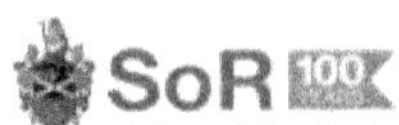

If you have or wear any of these, just let us know beforehand:

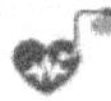 **Internal medical device** (e.g. pacemakers or orthopedic pins)

 **Hearing aids**

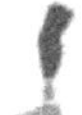 **Artificial limbs**

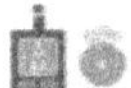 **Diabetic monitoring device**

 **RF ankle bracelets**

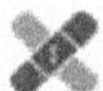 **Silver backed wound dressings**

 **Medicine patches** (e.g. HRT or Fentanyl)

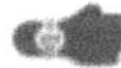 In-patient ID bracelets

 **Micro-bladed eyebrows**

 **Dental braces**

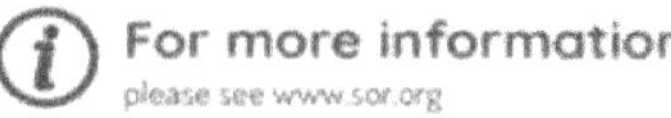

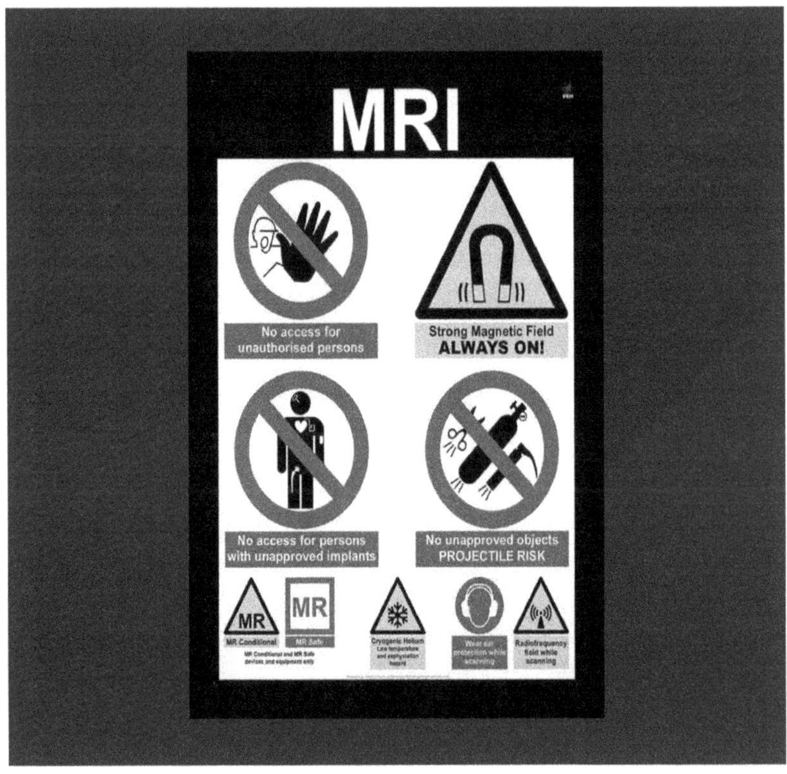
MRI
No access for
unauthorised persons
Strong Magnetic Field
ALWAYS ON!
No access for persons
with unapproved implants
No unapproved objects
PROJECTILE RISK
MR
MR
MR Conditional
MR Safe
MR Conditional and MR Safe
devices and equipment only
Cryogenic Helium
Low temperature
and asphyxiation
hazard
Wear ear
protection while
scanning
Radiofrequency
field while
scanning

CHAPTER 9

INTERVENTIONAL RADIOLOGY (IR)

Here's a chapter of the book on "Interventional Radiology" made Easy for Common People.

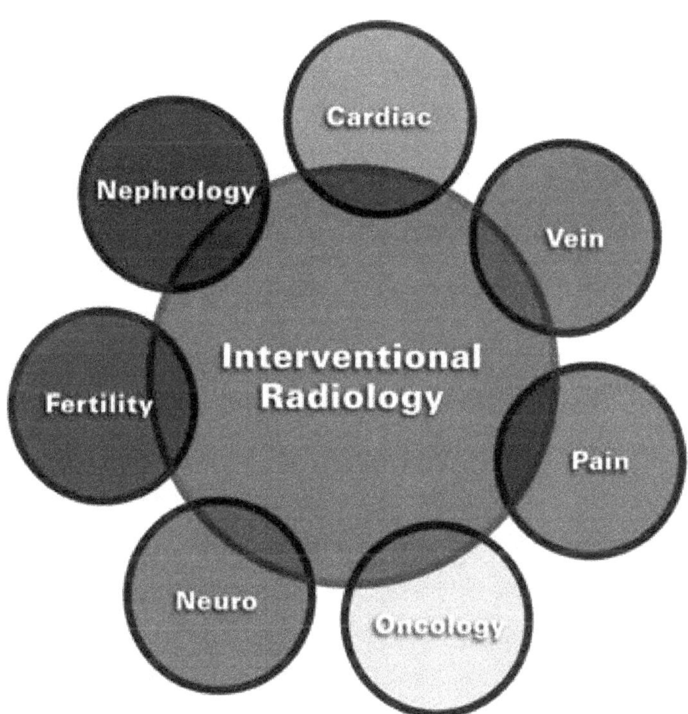

1. **What is Interventional Radiology?**

   - **Simple Definition**: Interventional radiology is a branch of radiology that uses imaging techniques (like X-rays, CT scans, ultrasound) to guide small tools and instruments inside the body for treatment. It is often a less invasive alternative to surgery.

- **Key Idea**: It helps doctors see inside the body and fix problems without making large cuts.

2. **How Does it Work?**

- **Imaging Techniques**: Explain the different imaging techniques used in interventional radiology:
  - **X-rays**: Highlight how they create images of bones and organs.
  - **CT scans**: Explain how they provide a detailed 3D view of the inside of the body.
  - **Ultrasound**: Illustrate how sound waves are used to see tissues in real-time.
- **Guided Procedures**: Describe how doctors use these images to guide tools like catheters (thin tubes) and wires to the affected area.

3. **Common Procedures in IR**

- **Angioplasty**: Explain how doctors open blocked blood vessels using a balloon.
- **Stent Placement**: Describe how tiny metal tubes (stents) are used to keep blood vessels open.
- **Biopsies**: Simplify how doctors can take small samples from tumors or organs without surgery.

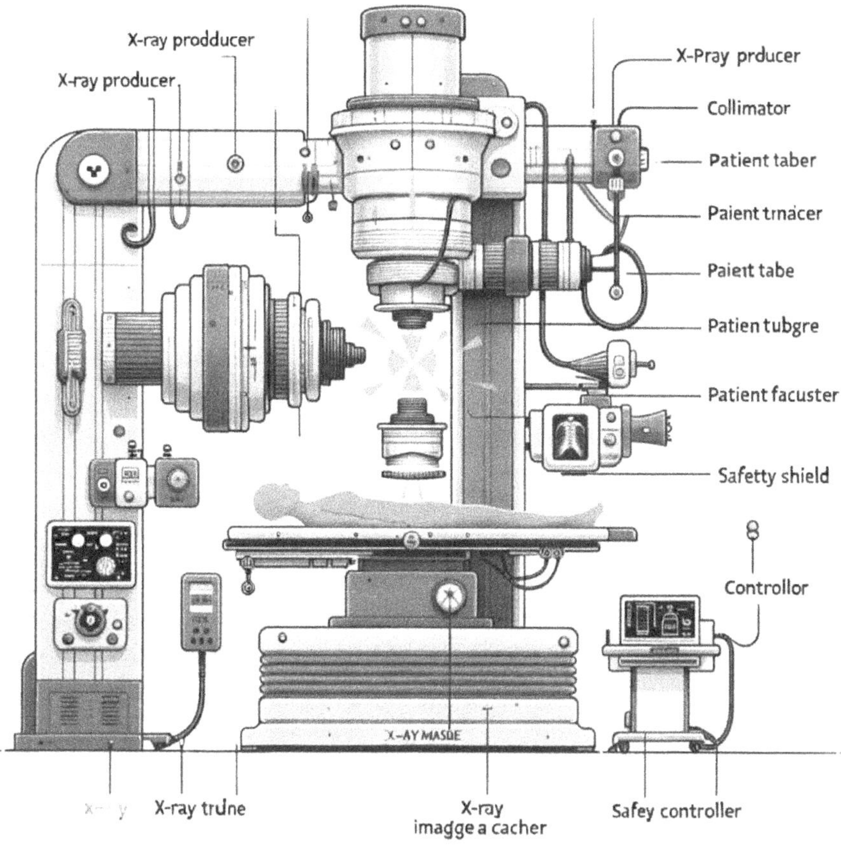

- **Embolization**: Show how doctors block blood flow to areas like tumors to reduce their size or stop bleeding.
- **Drainage of Fluids**: Discuss how abscesses or collections of fluid can be drained without needing large incisions.

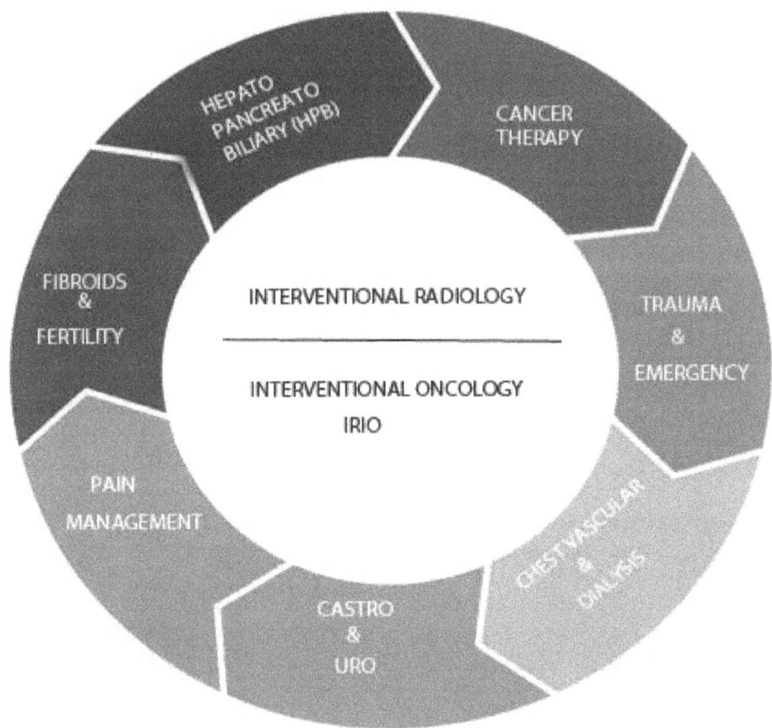

4. **Why Choose Interventional Radiology?**

   - **Less Invasive**: Explain how it usually requires only a small cut or puncture, leading to quicker recovery.
   - **Less Pain and Scarring**: Highlight that it causes less discomfort compared to traditional surgery.
   - **Faster Recovery**: Illustrate how people can often go home the same day or recover faster.

5. **Who Benefits from IR?**

   - Describe how interventional radiology is used for various conditions like:
     - **Cancer**: Treating tumors or providing pain relief.

    - **Vascular Problems**: Addressing blocked arteries or veins.
    - **Kidney and Liver Diseases**: Performing biopsies or draining blocked ducts.

6. **What Happens During a Procedure?**
    - **Before the Procedure**: Consultation process, how the patient is prepared, and what to expect.
    - **During the Procedure**: Simplify the steps, showing how the doctor uses imaging to guide instruments.
    - **After the Procedure**: Describe the recovery process and what patients should expect post-procedure.

7. **Myths and Misconceptions About Interventional Radiology**
    - **Myth**: "It's experimental and unsafe."
        - **Truth**: Explain that IR is a well-established, safe medical practice.
    - **Myth**: "It's only for rare conditions."
        - **Truth**: Show how it's widely used for common issues like blocked arteries or kidney problems.

8. **Real-Life Stories**

    Here are some real-life stories of common people explaining the advantages they've experienced through interventional radiology:

1. **Savita's story : Treatment for Uterine Fibroids**

    42-year-old woman from small village, had been suffering from painful uterine fibroids for years. She was apprehensive about undergoing a hysterectomy, fearing the long recovery time and potential impact on her quality of life. After a consultation, her doctor suggested **Uterine Fibroid Embolization (UFE)**, a minimally invasive procedure offered through interventional radiology.

Advantages:

- The procedure was done through a small incision in her wrist, and Savita was able to return home the same day.
- Her recovery took just a few days, compared to the weeks of recovery from a hysterectomy.
- Her symptoms improved significantly, and she was able to keep her uterus intact, something important to her overall well-being.

Savita said, "I couldn't believe how easy it was. I was back to work within a week, and I felt like I had my life back."

2. **Mallangouda Story: Angioplasty for Peripheral Artery Disease (PAD)**

   60-year-old retired teacher, was diagnosed with **Peripheral Artery Disease**. He had been experiencing severe leg pain that made walking difficult. His doctor recommended a minimally invasive angioplasty procedure, where interventional radiologists would insert a tiny balloon to open his clogged arteries.

Advantages:

- The procedure took just a couple of hours, and Mark only had a small puncture in his leg.
- He went home the same day and was able to walk without pain shortly after.

- Mark avoided the risks and long recovery associated with traditional bypass surgery.

He shared, “I expected to be laid up for weeks, but I was back on my feet the next day. It was life-changing.”

3. **Pooja Story: Cancer Treatment with Radiofrequency Ablation (RFA)** 55-year-old, was diagnosed with liver cancer. Instead of undergoing major surgery, her oncologist suggested **Radiofrequency Ablation (RFA)**, an IR procedure that uses heat to destroy cancer cells.

Advantages:

- The procedure was performed with a needle-like probe inserted through her skin, avoiding the need for large incisions.
- Pooja was able to go home the same day, with only minor discomfort.
- The tumor was successfully treated without the long recovery that traditional surgery would have required.

“It felt like a miracle. I was able to spend more time with my family during treatment instead of being in a hospital,” Pooja said.

4. **Jalindhar Story: Minimally Invasive Treatment for Varicose Veins**

   A 48-year-old construction worker, had been suffering from painful and unsightly varicose veins for years. He finally decided to undergo **Endovenous Laser Treatment (EVLT)**, a procedure in which a laser fiber is used to close off the problematic vein.

Advantages:

- The procedure was quick, requiring just a small puncture rather than large surgical cuts.
- John was able to resume light activity almost immediately, with no need for hospitalization.
- The pain in his legs diminished significantly, and the visible veins disappeared over time.

5. **Lina's Story: Treatment for Deep Vein Thrombosis (DVT)**

   Lina , a 33-year-old mother of two, developed **Deep Vein Thrombosis (DVT)** after a long flight. Instead of going through invasive surgery, her doctors recommended **Catheter-Directed Thrombolysis**, an IR procedure to dissolve the blood clot.

Advantages:

- The procedure was performed using a small catheter, minimizing the risk of bleeding and infection.
- Lina was able to return to her normal activities quickly, avoiding a lengthy hospital stay.
- The clot was dissolved, and she avoided potential complications like a pulmonary embolism.

"I felt so relieved that they could treat the clot without major surgery. I was back with my kids before I knew it," Lina recalled.

Few informative Illustrations and Diagrams

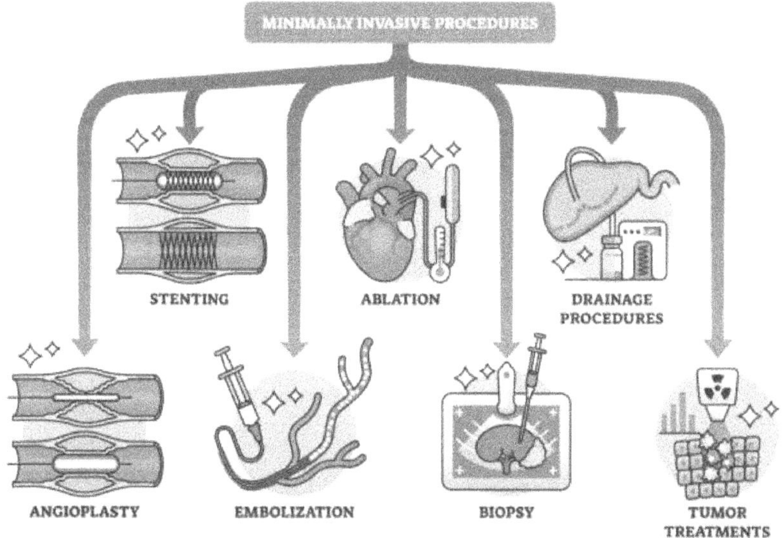

CONCLUSION :

1. **Greeting and Introduction**

- **Radiologist's Opening Statement**:
    - Start with a friendly and approachable tone.
    - Introduce yourself and your role: "Hello, I'm Dr. [Name], one of the radiologists who reviewed your recent [X-ray, CT, MRI, etc.]. My job is to look at the images and provide a clear understanding of what they show."
- **Patient's Information Confirmation**:
    - Confirm the patient's identity to ensure accurate communication: "Before we begin, can I confirm your

name and the date of the exam to make sure we're looking at the right information?"

2. **Explanation of the Imaging Study**
   - **Radiologist's Brief Overview**:
     - Give a simple explanation of the type of imaging study performed: "You had a [CT scan, MRI, ultrasound] of the [specific area] to help us investigate [the symptom or medical issue]."
   - **Purpose of the Exam**:
     - Provide context for the imaging study: "This type of scan is useful because it helps us get a clear view of the [bones, soft tissues, organs] in that area and identify any issues that may not be visible otherwise."
3. **Sharing Results**
   - **Use Clear, Non-Technical Language**:
     - Start by explaining whether the findings are normal or if there are any areas of concern: "The good news is that everything looks normal," or "We did find something that we want to explain further."
     - If there's an abnormality, describe it in simple terms: "We saw a small spot on your lung, which could be a number of things, like an infection or something less serious, but we want to follow up to be sure."
   - **Use Visual Aids**:
     - If possible, offer to show the patient the images: "Would you like me to show you the images and explain what you're seeing?"

   - Point out key areas on the image, using simple comparisons (e.g., "This dark area is the bone, and this lighter part is the soft tissue around it.")

4. **Clarifying the Diagnosis or Next Steps**

- **Explain What the Findings Mean**:
   - Avoid overwhelming the patient with too many details. Instead, focus on the key takeaway

CHAPTER 10

UNDERSTANDING PET-CT: A WINDOW INTO THE BODY'S FUNCTION AND HEALTH

Imagine your body as a bustling city. Roads connect different areas (organs), vehicles move along these roads (blood), and certain buildings (cells) are constantly working, consuming energy, and producing waste. Now, if something goes wrong, like a power outage in one part of the city (disease in the body), wouldn't it be helpful to know where the problem is and how severe it is? That's where a PET-CT scan steps in—a powerful imaging tool that helps doctors visualize not just the structure of your body but also its ongoing activities.

What is a PET-CT Scan?

- **PET (Positron Emission Tomography):** This part of the scan looks at how your cells are functioning. It detects areas in your body where cells are unusually active, which can indicate diseases like cancer, inflammation, or infections.
- **CT (Computed Tomography):** This part provides a detailed map of the body's structure, like a 3D blueprint of your organs, bones, and tissues.
- When combined, **PET-CT** creates a comprehensive image that shows both what your body looks like and how it's working, all in one scan.

How Does It Work?

Preparation: Before the scan, you're given a small amount of a radioactive substance (called a tracer) through an injection. Don't worry—this is safe and contains minimal radiation.

The most common tracer is a sugar-like molecule called **FDG (fluorodeoxyglucose)**. Since active cells (like cancer cells) consume more sugar, they "light up" on the scan.

Scanning Process:

- You lie down on a table that slides into a donut-shaped machine.
- The CT scan captures detailed images of your body's anatomy.
- The PET scan detects the tracer and highlights areas of abnormal activity.

Results: The images from the PET and CT are merged to give doctors a clearer picture of what's happening in your body.

When is a PET-CT Used?

Doctors recommend PET-CT for various reasons, including:

- **Cancer Detection and Staging:** Identifying tumors, determining their size, and checking if they've spread.
- **Treatment Monitoring:** Evaluating how well cancer treatment (like chemotherapy) is working.
- **Heart Problems:** Assessing blood flow to the heart or damage after a heart attack.

- **Brain Disorders:** Detecting conditions like Alzheimer's disease or epilepsy.

Why is PET-CT Important?

- It helps **diagnose diseases early**, often before symptoms appear.
- It provides precise information for **personalized treatment plans**.
- It reduces the need for invasive procedures like surgeries or biopsies.

What Should You Know Before a PET-CT Scan?

- **Fasting:** You may need to avoid eating for several hours before the scan.
- **Stay Still:** During the scan, it's essential to lie still for accurate images.
- **Safety:** The amount of radiation used is small and leaves your body quickly.

An Everyday Example

Think of a PET-CT like a weather radar for your body. The CT part shows the landscape—mountains, rivers, and cities (organs and tissues). The PET part shows where storms (disease) are brewing, even if they're not visible yet. Together, they help your doctor plan the "best route" to keep your body healthy.

Key Takeaway

PET-CT is a groundbreaking tool that combines the power of seeing your body's structure and understanding its function.

Whether it's spotting disease early, planning treatment, or tracking progress, PET-CT helps doctors unlock the secrets of your body's inner workings—helping you stay on the path to better health.

CHAPTER 11

HOW RADIOLOGISTS DIAGNOSE?

Radiologists use various clues in medical images to aid in diagnosis, combining their knowledge of anatomy, pathology, and imaging technology to interpret what they see. Here's how radiologists use these clues to make accurate diagnoses:

1. **Understanding Normal Anatomy**

   - **Clue**: Before identifying abnormalities, radiologists must know what healthy organs, tissues, and structures look like on different imaging modalities (X-rays, CT, MRI, ultrasound, etc.).
   - **Use**: They compare the patient's images to this baseline of normal anatomy, looking for anything unusual in size, shape, or texture.

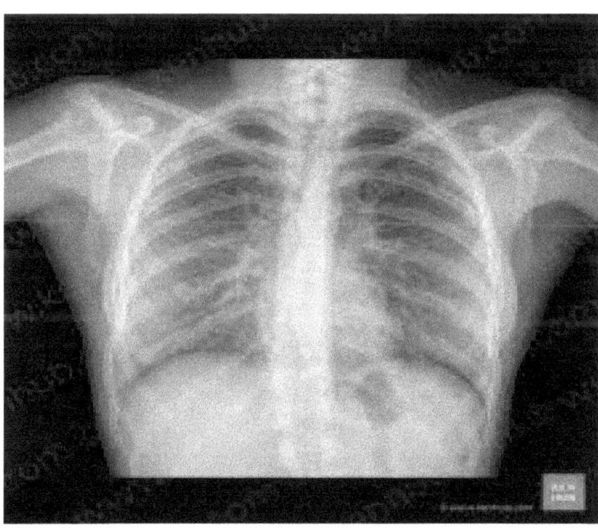

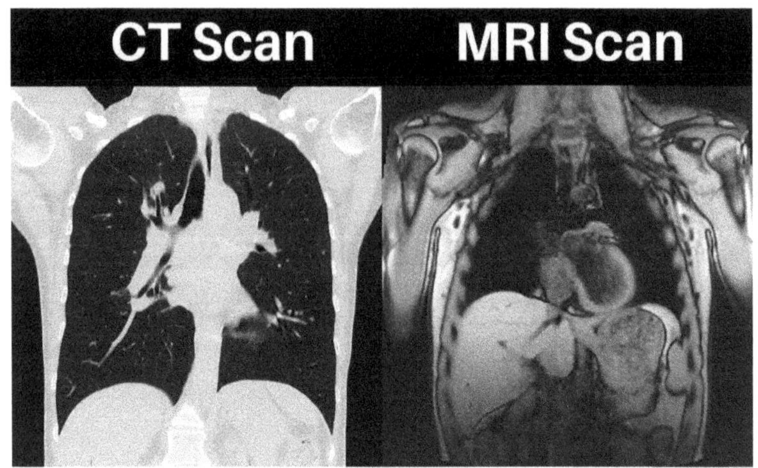

NORMAL RADIOLOGICAL PICTURES OF CHEST ON X RAY, CT AND MRI.

X RAY – 2D IMAGE GROSS OVERVIEW

CT – BEST FOR LUNG, BONE & HEART RELATED PATHOLOHY

MRI – SOFT TISSUE , MUSCLE, HEART AND CHEST WALL

2. **Identifying Patterns**

- **Clue**: Certain diseases or conditions create recognizable patterns in medical images.
- **Use**: Radiologists are trained to recognize these patterns and match them to specific conditions. For example:
    - **Lung Diseases**: Pneumonia shows up on a chest X-ray as patchy white areas (consolidations) in the lung, while lung cancer may present as a solitary, irregular mass.

- **Fractures**: Bone fractures are typically seen as dark lines where the bone has broken on X-rays.
- **Brain Abnormalities**: A stroke on a CT scan can appear as a darker (or lighter) area due to disrupted blood flow, while an MRI may show more detailed tissue damage.

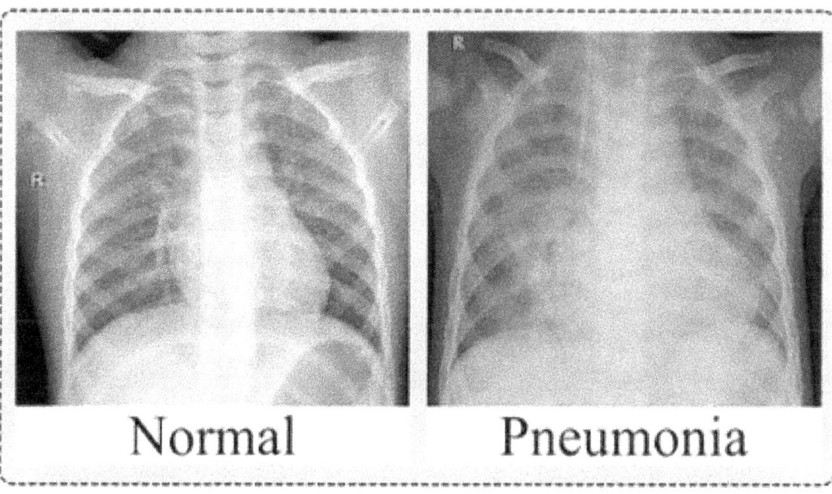

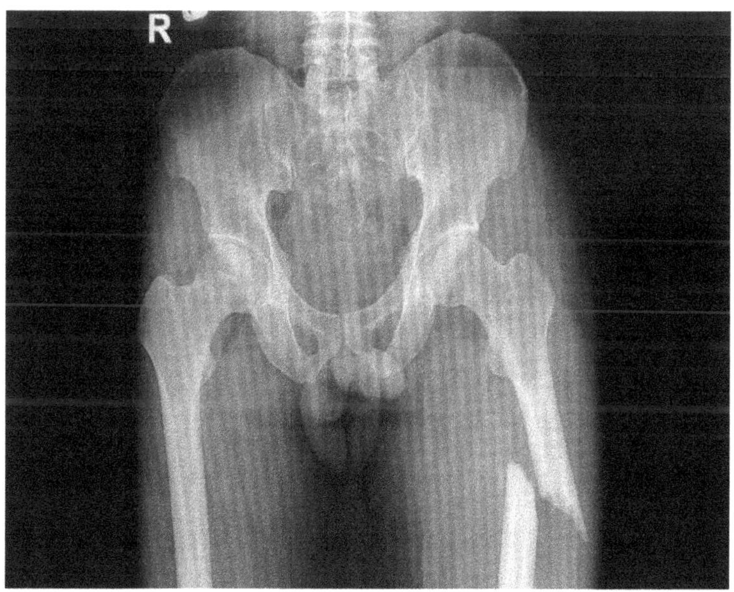

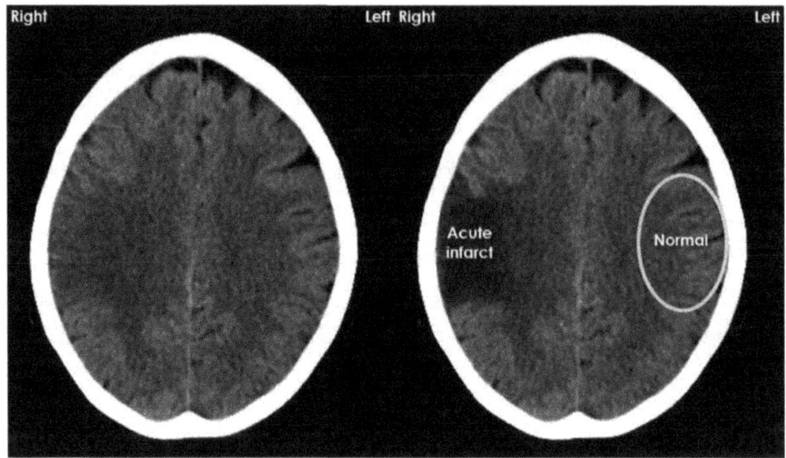

3. **Evaluating Density and Signal Intensity**

   - **Clue**: The density or brightness (signal intensity) of tissues varies between healthy and diseased states, depending on the imaging modality used.
   - **Use**:
     - **X-rays and CT Scans**: Denser materials like bone appear white, while air or fluid appears darker.
     - **MRI**: Different tissues emit different signals in MRI, with fat appearing bright and water appearing dark in certain sequences. Tumors often have different signal intensities compared to surrounding healthy tissue, helping to differentiate them.

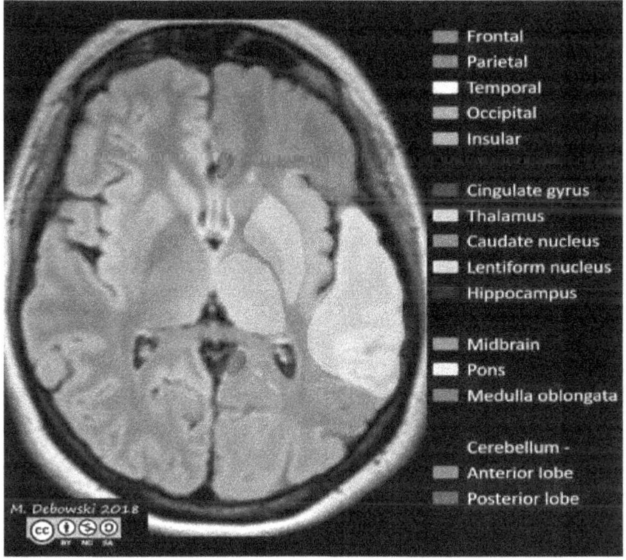

4. **Spotting Changes in Size or Shape**

   - **Clue**: Changes in the size or shape of organs or structures can signal disease.
   - **Use**:
     - **Heart and Lungs**: An enlarged heart on a chest X-ray may indicate heart failure, while a rounded, swollen lung border may suggest pleural effusion (fluid around the lungs).
     - **Tumor Growth**: Enlarged lymph nodes or growths in organs like the liver or kidneys can indicate the presence of tumors or cancer.

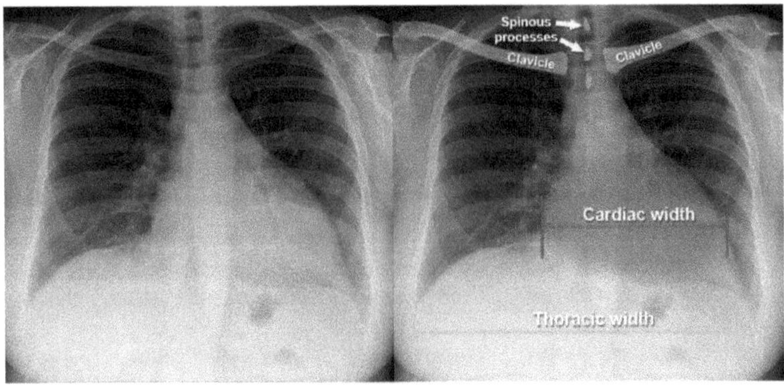

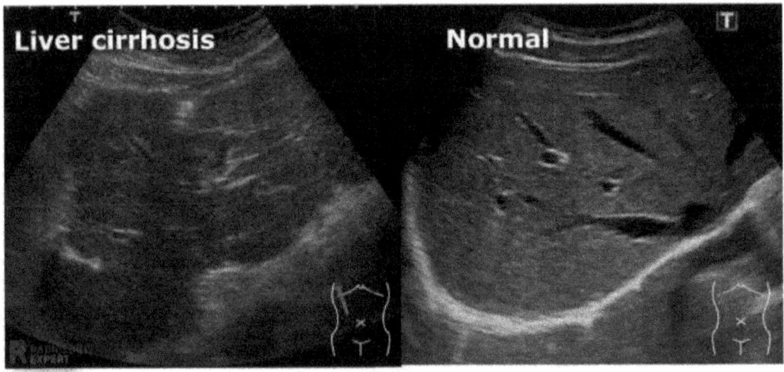

5. **Looking for Contrast Enhancement**

- **Clue**: Radiologists often use contrast agents (e.g., iodine or gadolinium) in CT or MRI scans to highlight certain structures or abnormalities.
- **Use**: Contrast helps differentiate between different types of tissue or abnormalities:
  - **Tumors**: Many tumors "light up" or enhance after contrast is administered, showing more clearly compared to normal tissue.

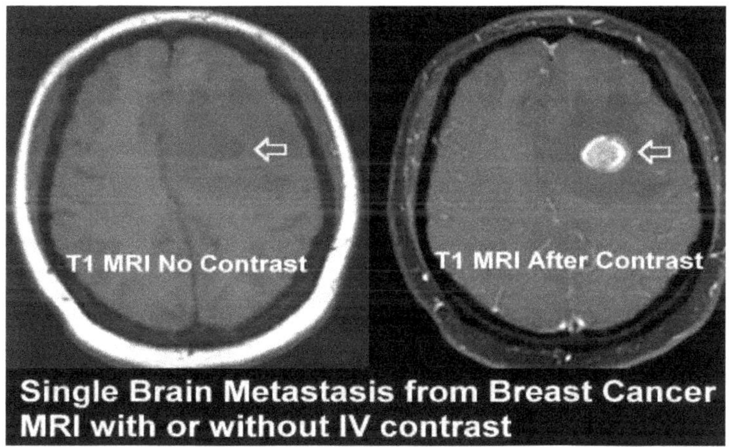

Single Brain Metastasis from Breast Cancer
MRI with or without IV contrast

6. **Analyzing Symmetry**
   - **Clue**: Healthy anatomy is typically symmetrical on both sides of the body.
   - **Use**: Radiologists look for asymmetry to detect abnormalities:
     - **Breasts**: In mammography, asymmetry between the two breasts can suggest a mass or abnormal growth.
     - **Brain**: In brain imaging, asymmetry might indicate a stroke, tumor, or injury affecting one side of the brain.

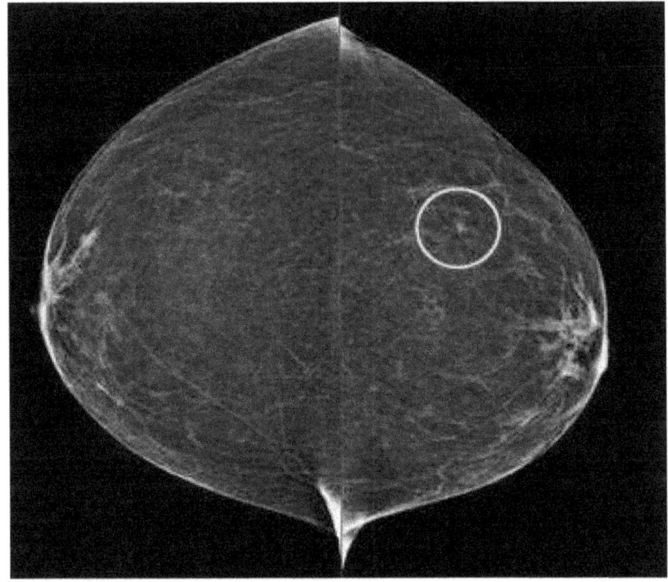

7. **Assessing Organ Function**

- **Clue**: Some imaging modalities, like PET scans or functional MRIs (fMRI), assess organ function rather than just structure.
- **Use**: Radiologists look for areas with abnormal metabolism or blood flow:
    - **Cancer**: PET scans detect areas of high glucose uptake, which often indicates cancer, as tumors usually consume more energy.
    - **Brain Function**: fMRI measures brain activity by detecting changes in blood flow, which can help in diagnosing conditions like epilepsy or evaluating the effects of a stroke.

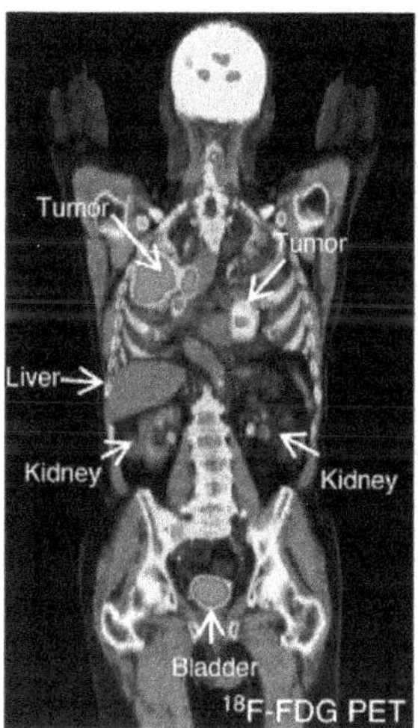

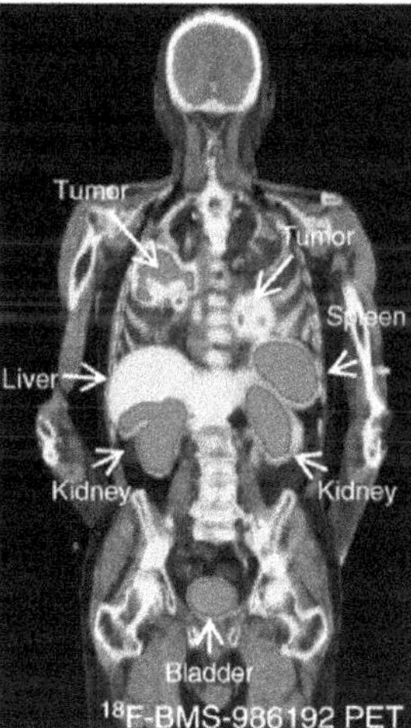

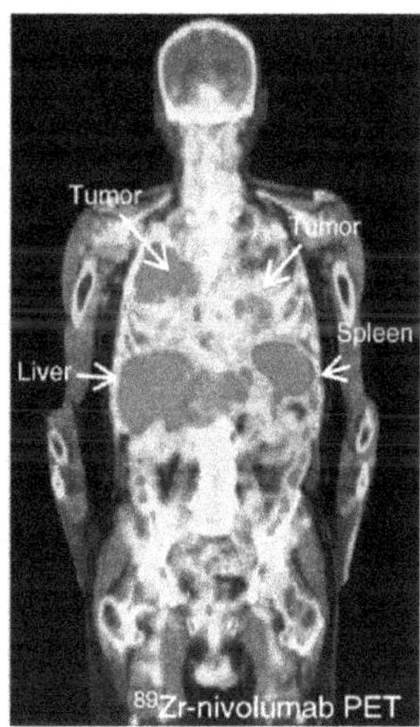

8. **Detecting Calcifications**

   - **Clue**: Calcifications (deposits of calcium) can appear as bright, white spots on X-rays, CTs, or mammograms.
   - **Use**: These can be a sign of certain conditions:
     - **Breast Cancer**: Microcalcifications in the breast can be an early sign of breast cancer, while larger calcifications are often benign.
     - **Atherosclerosis**: Calcifications in the arteries may indicate plaque buildup, which can lead to heart disease or stroke.

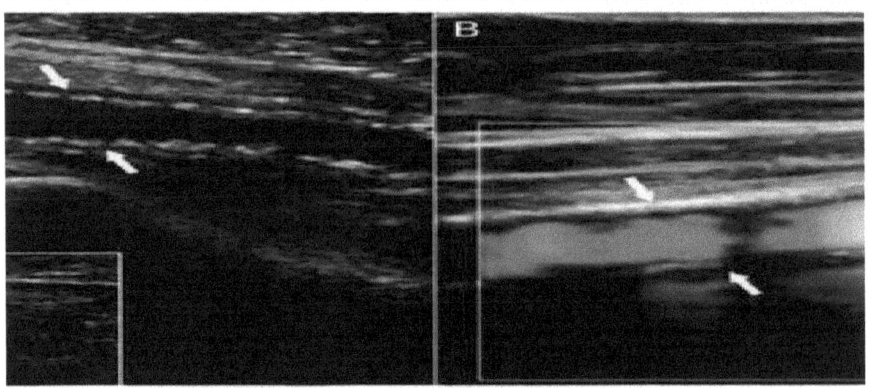

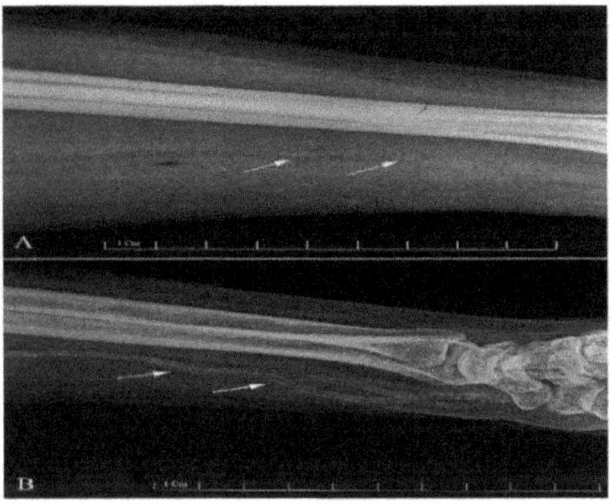

9. **Correlating with Clinical Information**

    - **Clue**: Radiologists don't work in isolation—they combine imaging findings with clinical information from the patient's history, symptoms, and lab results.
    - **Use**: For example, if a patient presents with severe abdominal pain and a CT scan shows inflammation around the appendix, the radiologist can confidently diagnose appendicitis. Without clinical context, the same inflammation could be mistaken for something else.

10. **Using Prior Imaging for Comparison**

- **Clue**: Changes over time can provide important diagnostic clues.
- **Use**: Radiologists often compare new scans with older ones to see how a condition is progressing:
  - **Cancer**: A shrinking tumor may indicate successful treatment, while a growing one suggests the cancer is worsening.
  - **Bone Healing**: In cases of fractures, radiologists assess how well bones are healing over time.

Summary:

Radiologists use a combination of anatomical knowledge, pattern recognition, density analysis, symmetry checks, and clinical correlation to make accurate diagnoses. By carefully studying these clues in medical images, they can provide critical information to help doctors make informed decisions about patient care.

CONCLUSION: DEMYSTIFYING RADIOLOGY FOR EVERYONE

Radiology is more than just pictures; it's a window into the human body, offering invaluable insights that guide diagnosis and treatment.

From X-rays to MRIs, CT scans to ultrasounds, each tool has its unique strengths and applications.

As we conclude, remember that being an informed patient is one of the best ways to actively participate in your health journey. Understanding imaging tests and their purposes can reduce anxiety, improve communication with your medical team, and ultimately enhance your overall healthcare experience.

Thank you for taking the time to learn about radiology. It's my hope that this knowledge not only answers your questions but also inspires you to share this understanding with others, helping to make radiology accessible to all.

After all, knowledge is power—and in healthcare, it can also be healing.

Stay curious, stay informed and take charge of your health.

Radiology has unveiled its secrets; now it's up to you to use this knowledge wisely!

www.ingramcontent.com/pod-product-compliance
Lightning Source LLC
LaVergne TN
LVHW021157160826
845679LV00024B/2143